Understanding Human Metabolism

Does eating more carbohydrates, or fats, cause one to put on more weight? Are ketone bodies toxins or vital products that keep us alive during starvation? Does the concept of 'fat-burning exercise' hold true? In this game-changing book, Keith Frayn, an international expert in human metabolism and nutrition, dispels common misconceptions about human metabolism, explaining in everyday language the important metabolic processes that underlie all aspects of our daily lives. Illustrated throughout with clear diagrams of metabolic processes, Frayn describes the communication systems that enable our different organs and tissues to cooperate, for instance in providing fuel to our muscles when we exercise, and in preserving our tissues during fasting. He explores the impressive adaptability of human metabolism and discusses the metabolic disorders that can arise when metabolism 'goes wrong.' For anyone sceptical of information about diet and lifestyle, this concise book guides the reader through what metabolism really involves.

Keith Frayn is Emeritus Professor of Human Metabolism at the University of Oxford, UK. In a long and varied career studying human metabolism and nutrition, he has worked in various settings, from diabetes clinics to Accident and Emergency departments and Intensive Care wards. His work has been widely recognised with awards including the first Blaxter Medal of the Nutrition Society, the David Cuthbertson Lecture at the European Society of Parenteral and Enteral Nutrition, and Honorary Fellowship of the Nutrition Society.

The *Understanding Life* series is for anyone wanting an engaging and concise way into a key biological topic. Offering a multidisciplinary perspective, these accessible guides address common misconceptions and misunderstandings in a thoughtful way to help stimulate debate and encourage a more in-depth understanding. Written by leading thinkers in each field, these books are for anyone wanting an expert overview that will enable clearer thinking on each topic.

Series Editor: Kostas Kampourakis http://kampourakis.com

Published titles:

Understanding Evolution	Kostas Kampourakis	9781108746083
Understanding Coronavirus	Raul Rabadan	9781108826716
Understanding Development	Alessandro Minelli	9781108799232
Understanding Evo-Devo	Wallace Arthur	9781108819466
Understanding Genes	Kostas Kampourakis	9781108812825
Understanding DNA Ancestry	Sheldon Krimsky	9781108816038
Understanding Intelligence	Ken Richardson	9781108940368
Understanding Metaphors in the Life Sciences	Andrew S. Reynolds	9781108940498
Understanding Cancer	Robin Hesketh	9781009005999
Understanding How Science Explains the World	Kevin McCain	9781108995504
Understanding Race	Rob DeSalle and Ian Tattersall	9781009055581
Understanding Human Evolution	Ian Tattersall	9781009101998
Understanding Human Metabolism	Keith N. Frayn	9781009108522

Forthcoming:

Understanding Fertility	Gab Kovacs	9781009054164
Understanding Forensic DNA	Suzanne Bell and John M. Butler	9781009044011
Understanding Natural Selection	Michael Ruse	9781009088329
Understanding Life in the Universe	Wallace Arthur	9781009207324

Understanding Human Metabolism

KEITH N. FRAYN
Emeritus Professor of Human Metabolism, University of Oxford

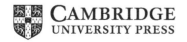

CAMBRIDGE
UNIVERSITY PRESS

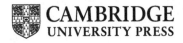

CAMBRIDGE
UNIVERSITY PRESS

Shaftesbury Road, Cambridge CB2 8EA, United Kingdom

One Liberty Plaza, 20th Floor, New York, NY 10006, USA

477 Williamstown Road, Port Melbourne, VIC 3207, Australia

314–321, 3rd Floor, Plot 3, Splendor Forum, Jasola District Centre, New Delhi – 110025, India

103 Penang Road, #05–06/07, Visioncrest Commercial, Singapore 238467

Cambridge University Press is part of Cambridge University Press & Assessment,
a department of the University of Cambridge.

We share the University's mission to contribute to society through the pursuit of
education, learning and research at the highest international levels of excellence.

www.cambridge.org
Information on this title: www.cambridge.org/9781009108522

DOI: 10.1017/9781009104463

First published 2022

A catalogue record for this publication is available from the British Library

Library of Congress Cataloging-in-Publication data
Names: Frayn, K. N. (Keith N.), author.
Title: Understanding human metabolism / Keith N. Frayn, Emeritus of the University of Oxford.
Description: First edition. | Cambridge, United Kingdom; New York, NY: Cambridge University Press, 2022. |
    Series: ULF understanding life | Includes bibliographical references and index.
Identifiers: LCCN 2022970034 (print) | LCCN 2022970035 (ebook) | ISBN 9781009100076 (hardback) |
    ISBN 9781009108522 (paperback) | ISBN 9781009104463 (epub)
Subjects: LCSH: Metabolism. | Obesity–Endocrine aspect.
Classification: LCC QP171 .F735 2022 (print) | LCC QP171 (ebook) | DDC 612.3/9–dc23/eng/20220330
LC record available at https://lccn.loc.gov/2022970034
LC ebook record available at https://lccn.loc.gov/2022970035

ISBN   978-1-009-10007-6   Hardback
ISBN   978-1-009-10852-2   Paperback

Are you interested in your health and want to understand how your body functions? Do you want to learn the science behind how food and exercise interact and how together they can both foster wellbeing or lead to poor health and disease? This, and all you need to know about the key role of human metabolism for health and disease, is what *Understanding Human Metabolism* gives you. The author, Professor Keith Frayn, is probably the best teacher of human metabolism and nutrition of our times and has published several superb books on the topic for students of medicine and nutrition. This time, I would like to congratulate anyone without medical training but with an interest in human metabolism – this is *the* book for you.

> Olle Ljungqvist, Professor of Surgery, Örebro University and
> Affiliated Professor of Surgery, Nutrition and Metabolism,
> Karolinska Institute, Sweden

Insightful, objective, easy reading. Nutritional biochemistry and metabolism in the right measure.

> Teresa H M da Costa, Professor, Department of Nutrition,
> University of Brasília, Brazil

Everyone has a metabolism, and most people have a folk understanding of it. This very clear account of this actually complex subject brings science to bear on such understandings. Reading it will help you understand yourself better.

> Stanley Ulijaszek, Professor of Human Ecology,
> University of Oxford, UK

Contents

Foreword

Metabolism. A term that many people have heard of, but also one that very few would be able to define correctly. Among those who would be able to provide a definition, most would end up using terms from biochemistry such as glycolysis, Krebs cycle, and oxidative phosphorylation, remembering the hard time they had learning all these biochemical reactions and pathways at some point during their studies. This might make you wonder then if the concept of metabolism, and whatever it is about, has any relevance to your everyday life. Well, in this splendid book, Keith Frayn tells you that it does – and why it does. More than this, he explains to you what metabolism is, and that all these reactions and pathways are relevant to your everyday life. Understanding them will make you get a sense of what is going on inside our bodies when we eat food, as well as when we do not; why we may be fatter or thinner than we would have wanted to be; and why sugars and lipids are not bad for us but essential for our life. By describing research on these topics over several decades, Frayn also explains how we came to understand metabolism, and figure out many of the complex ways that our organs are interrelated and interdependent. Reading this book is a rewarding experience, as a lot that you have heard of will suddenly make sense. Frayn paints a beautiful picture that will help you understand why we eat what we eat, what happens to that once we eat it, and how our bodies have evolved to be able to adjust to what is available to eat. In today's societies in which food tends to be plentiful, this might sound irrelevant. Well, I would argue that exactly because food tends to be plentiful, understanding metabolism is crucial for being able to make appropriate and balanced choices regarding what to eat.

Kostas Kampourakis, Series Editor

Preface

Surely not another book about metabolism? I can almost hear it being said. There seems to be a plethora of books at present about how to prevent oneself becoming obese, how to lose weight if one has already become so, what one should eat, and especially what one should not eat. There are books about the importance, or otherwise, of exercise for maintaining weight and health, and books about how to live longer by eating the diet of our palaeolithic ancestors or our near-relations in the animal world.

But none of these really addresses the field that biochemists know as intermediary metabolism. That term refers to the chemical processes that occur within our bodies – mostly within our cells – that transform what we eat into useful energy, new bodily constituents, and waste products. Indeed, from a reading of current popular science on the topic of metabolism, you might well have the impression that 'metabolism' refers just to the 'burning' of foodstuffs with the result either of weight loss or weight gain. You would not then appreciate the myriad of chemical reactions that build up the substances of which we are made, break them down again when they are no longer needed, and create safely disposable waste products. Even our DNA, the material of which our genes is made, is formed from chemical building blocks that are the product of such reactions.

Many features of intermediary metabolism must have evolved a very long time ago, since they are common to all life forms – from bacteria to mammals (Chapter 1). But it seems natural for us to have a particular interest in our own metabolism – human metabolism. And there is good reason for that. What goes on inside us is a product not just of chemical reactions, but of a flow of information between different body parts regulating just what happens and when – so that when I have just eaten a big meal, my cells begin to store nutrients, and when I have not eaten for some time, they will begin to release nutrients from these stores (Chapters 2 and 3). Such information flow, called metabolic regulation, is a product largely of our hormonal and nervous systems (Chapter 4).

If there is one feature of intermediary, or cellular, metabolism that is widely known it is perhaps the so-called Krebs cycle, more commonly called by scientists the citric acid cycle, discovered by Hans Krebs (later Professor Sir Hans Krebs). But even those who know the term may well not appreciate just what this assembly of chemical reactions does. It can be seen as the 'final common pathway' by which all nutrients are broken down, and linked to the release of energy in a form that can be used by cells for all the processes that require it (Chapter 5).

The really wonderful – and often not appreciated – feature of our metabolism is that it is active, and changing, all the time: when you eat breakfast after fasting overnight, metabolism changes quickly; when you start to exercise, it changes even more quickly. During a typical day, chemical reactions in our cells are being accelerated and slowed down in a highly coordinated manner, enabling us to continue leading our daily lives without giving this matter any thought whatsoever (Chapter 6). But I rather hope that, once you understand what these changes entail, you might think about them more than you probably do at present. Changes in metabolism, as just noted, are especially marked during exercise, when our muscles require a supply of energy, that may come from within the muscles' own cells, or may be brought in the blood from other tissues, especially our fat stores and our liver. However we measure 'metabolism', there is no doubt that it is going faster when we are exercising than when we are at rest. But the opposite is true in starvation. When the body is deprived of nutrients, then metabolism is suppressed, conserving the precious stores that we have of metabolic fuels. Our carbohydrate stores are especially precious, the proteins of which our bodies are mostly built even more so, and metabolic mechanisms come into play to preserve these for as long as possible whilst living off our usually plentiful fat stores. The way these changes are brought about in starvation and in exercise is a fascinating aspect of our metabolism that presumably evolved to allow our ancestors to chase, or run from, other animals, and to survive even when no food was forthcoming (Chapter 7).

There is a tendency nowadays to regard carbohydrates, fats, and proteins as separate entities which can each be considered in isolation. This cannot be the view of anyone who has seriously studied human metabolism. The metabolic fates of the three major energy-providing nutrients are, of necessity, intimately intertwined. Our bodies are all the time drawing upon individual nutrients for particular needs: indeed, each of our tissues has its own preferences for particular fuels at different times. And all these requirements must be coordinated. Metabolic scientists now understand many ways in which the metabolic fates of the nutrients inter-relate. At a very basic level, all energy-providing nutrients, including alcohol, feed into the same cellular mechanism for final disposal, the citric acid (or Krebs) cycle, mentioned earlier. They have to share this pathway, and, just like family members sharing a bathtub, they cannot all get in at once. In Chapter 8 we will look at the mechanisms that prevent overcrowding.

But of course, like any other finely tuned system, things can go wrong. Many diseases involve disturbances in one or more of the myriad of metabolic processes that keep us going. Some of these are inherited very directly from our parents. Others are the result of our environment, but most are a combination of both influences. There are fairly common examples of disorders in the metabolism of carbohydrates, fats, and proteins (or the amino acids that make up proteins), and there are more complex conditions that may involve all three, diabetes mellitus (commonly just called diabetes) being one of these. What is more, metabolic changes may underlie common diseases such as cardiovascular disease (e.g. heart attack, stroke) and even cancer (Chapter 9).

I consider myself very lucky to have been able to spend my career investigating something that I find so intensely interesting – human metabolism. About half-way through my career, I was tempted to write down my views of this field so I could 'spread the word'. The result was an undergraduate textbook, then called *Metabolic Regulation: A Human Perspective*. This book has proved to be popular for students and researchers in a variety of fields, and the current, fourth edition, is now called *Human Metabolism: A Regulatory Perspective* (written with R. D. Evans). But these books are not really 'popular science', as some reviews attest (e.g. '*Whoops! I requested this book not realising it was a textbook, I thought it would be a bit more (dare I say it?) dummed down. Not that I'm stupid, but this just isn't my field ....*'). So, this book, *Understanding Human Metabolism*, is now my attempt to present some of the wonder of human metabolism to a wider audience. My aims are twofold. Firstly, I would like others to share my amazement at this wonderful system, the result of millions of years of evolution, and underpinning our daily lives. But, secondly, I really do believe that if more people were to understand just how their metabolism works, we might hear less of the simplistic views on diet and lifestyle that are so often peddled in the media.

Acknowledgements

I would like to thank the many people who encouraged me to study human metabolism, and worked with me during my long career, but they are too numerous to list here. I would, though, like to mention those who sparked my interest in metabolism during my undergraduate years in Cambridge, especially Nick Hales and Philip Tubbs. I was lucky to have such inspiring lecturers at a time when molecular biology was in the ascendency. I really learned how to do human metabolic physiology during my years with the Medical Research Council's Trauma Unit in Manchester, with the help of Manchester colleagues (I thank especially Rod Little), under the head of the unit, H. B. Stoner. A number of clinical colleagues helped me adapt to research work in an emergency setting, David Yates (the first Professor of Emergency Medicine in the UK) especially. During this time, George Alberti, Roy Taylor, and others at the University of Newcastle upon Tyne were very supportive with my metabolic work and helped me to become a better scientist. In Oxford, my 'boss' for six years was Derek Hockaday, who had built up a unit with wonderful facilities for human physiology, and I am grateful to him for allowing me to pursue my own developing interests in fat metabolism and nutrition. I worked with many, many colleagues in Oxford but especial thanks are due to Barbara Fielding, Geoff Gibbons, Leanne Hodson, Sandy Humphreys, and Fredrik Karpe, with each of whom I worked very closely for a long time. Intensive Care doctor Rhys Evans has been a good colleague and in recent years a co-author. My apologies to all those whose names I haven't been able to list.

The impetus to write this book specifically came from Anna Whiting at Cambridge University Press when I approached her with various woolly ideas about writing something on metabolism. I am very grateful to Anna and her colleague Olivia Boult for steering me through the process, and to Kostas Kampourakis, the Series Editor, for his many insightful comments – in particular for his vigorous striking-out of any mention of 'purpose' in metabolism!

I am grateful to Fredrik Karpe and John Miller for sending me, and allowing me to use, data from the Oxford BioBank. Kiki Marinou read and helped me with the section on diabetic ketoacidosis, in which she has great clinical experience. Jenny Collins was happy for me to use ideas about 'metabolic channelling', discussed in Chapter 3, derived from her work with fat cells in my laboratory.

This is my first book aimed specifically at the non-scientist, and a number of people have helped me at various stages along the way by reading my drafts and steering me in the right direction, including my wife Theresa and my daughter Liz, and my friend Nick Havely of the University of York, an expert in fourteenth-century Italian, French, and English literature: a real test of my comprehensibility. I will dedicate this book, though, to my grandchildren, Rayya, Alastair, Jibreel, Daniel, and Laith, in the hope it may inspire them to an interest in science and medicine.

1 What Is Metabolism?

Metabolism Is a Very Big Subject

Everyone seems to know about metabolism.

If I let slip at a social occasion that my job is researching into human metabolism, there are not many people who will not express an interest. A typical conversation might be:

> ' ... oh, I do research into human metabolism.'
> 'Wow, that's so interesting!'
> 'Are you interested in metabolism, then?'
> 'Yes, can you explain why mine is so slow?'

Or, more rarely,

> 'Yes, can you explain why mine is so fast?'

But the idea that 'metabolism' is just concerned with how fast, or slowly, we might burn off excess energy is a very restricted one. A commentator announced recently on the radio that 'the economy has slowed by 30%' (as a result of the coronavirus pandemic). I suppose this refers to the Gross Domestic Product, GDP. But I don't know what things contribute to this, or how they interact and how each is regulated. My wife and I try to buy produce from local shops, thinking we are doing some good for 'the local economy'. I guess the overall economy is made up of many 'local economies', together with other things like, for instance, manufacturing and garbage disposal. If that is so, then there are many parallels with metabolism. I am guessing that my understanding of economics is very similar to most people's understanding of metabolism. Yes, there are ways of capturing an 'overall' figure for a person's metabolism, but that in turn is made up a myriad of smaller components. And we can't understand the 'overall' picture, let alone how it might change, without having some knowledge of these components that contribute to it.

Almost every component of our bodies is the result of a metabolic process. The DNA that constitutes our genes is made from smaller components, each of which can be manufactured in our cells. The proteins that make up much of our cells are made from amino acids: there are 20 common amino acids in our proteins, and a few that occur in smaller amounts. Many of these amino acids can be made in our cells from other components, or interconverted, and they can all be broken down in our cells in metabolic processes. These metabolic processes are covered in specialised textbooks of biochemistry, but clearly it would be impossible to cover them in a book of this size. The most active metabolic processes in our bodies, in terms of mass converted, are those involving the nutrients that we eat, and use as building material and to derive energy, and these are therefore the processes on which we shall concentrate our attention. I guess that for many readers it just so happens that these are the very metabolic processes that will be of most interest.

Metabolism Developed Very Early in Evolution

The basic features of human metabolism must have evolved very early in the evolution of life. Our metabolism shares many features with the most distantly related organisms, bacteria and yeasts for example. If you were to give me a yeast cell and a human cell and ask me to study them in the laboratory, I might struggle to tell them apart (without genetic sequencing or looking at them through a microscope) – unless the yeast cell happened to break down sugar to make alcohol, which would be a give-away (yeast cells convert sugar to alcohol in the process called fermentation). One common feature of most life forms is that energy produced from breaking down nutrients is not used immediately (e.g. for movement or growth), but is trapped in a compound called adenosine triphosphate – ATP. ATP is the universal 'energy currency' of life. In humans, as we shall see, most ATP is generated in a metabolic process called the citric acid cycle (or Krebs cycle, after its discoverer). Similar processes are found in all life forms, including bacteria. Undoubtedly, many aspects of metabolism were present in whatever early cells predated the split between bacteria and other life forms.

Clearly you are reading this book because you are interested in human metabolism, but should you, in the future, decide to become a plant scientist or to work on exotic marine organisms, or even bacteria, a lot of what we will cover together in this journey will still be very closely applicable.

Human Metabolism Must Depend upon a Flow of Information

We have seen the universality of the underlying pathways of cellular metabolism. (A metabolic pathway is a series of chemical reactions, each brought about by a specific protein [an enzyme], that has the effect of transforming one substance into another. We shall look at metabolic pathways in more detail in Chapter 3.) But the metabolic patterns of humans, indeed of all animals, have some distinct and some common features. Humans mostly have fairly regular patterns of fasting and feeding, not eating overnight and then taking in discrete meals during the day. We are not like smaller mammals, shrews for example, that need to eat pretty well all the time in order to provide enough energy to generate the heat that they need to survive. So it stands to reason that, after we have eaten, we have means to store nutrients beyond our immediate needs, and then to release them from these stores as needed.

Consider, for instance, what happens to the fat that we eat. We eat a juicy burger, maybe with some fries. There will be a lot more fat in that meal than we need for energy for several hours. There is a metabolic pathway that leads the excess fat into specialised cells, fat cells (called adipocytes), where it is stored. But overnight, when we don't have food available, we will need to draw on those stores. Should I decide to get up in the morning and jog before breakfast, I will still have plenty of energy available to do so: fat stored in my fat cells, and carbohydrates stored in my muscles and my liver. And, should I be out for a very long jog (and fail to take some nourishment with me), my liver can turn on a pathway to make more carbohydrate (glucose, in fact). We see that metabolic pathways – storage of fat, bringing fat out of its stores to be used, and similar pathways for carbohydrates – are not constant in time (as they might be in a bacterial cell, for instance): they are activated at certain times and suppressed at others. This is 'metabolic regulation' and is arguably the most interesting aspect of human metabolism.

Immediately we can see that humans, unlike bacteria, must have means of internal signalling, 'telling' metabolic processes when to become active and when to shut down. I want to go for a walk. My brain sends signals to my leg muscles telling them to move. My muscles need more energy, from fat stores in my fat cells and from carbohydrate stores in my liver. Signals have to travel around orchestrating these processes. As we shall see, both nerves and hormones play a role in such regulation, and we shall learn that hormones have quite remarkable powers of regulation over metabolic pathways.

Another difference from the pathways of cellular metabolism that a bacteriologist might study is that such pathways involve cooperation between different tissues and organs. Any one of my cells (I have maybe 30 trillion cells) cannot survive on its own for more than perhaps 24 hours if I try to culture it in a laboratory flask. But my body could survive a month or two of complete starvation – indeed, there are records of people surviving more than 3 months' starvation, that we shall look at later. This involves fuels being transferred around the body, changes in the pathways of metabolism to conserve reserves, and of course all coordinated by nerves and hormones. During exercise, fuels will need to be transferred to the muscles: there must be changes in blood flow to deliver fuels and oxygen to the muscles and remove waste products. These are essentially illustrations of what is called 'integrative physiology' – the opposite, in a way, of the reductionist approach of molecular biology that looks in smaller and smaller detail at what goes on within cells.

Integrative physiology has had a rough time in recent decades. Since I started to study biochemistry in the 1960s, many Nobel Prizes have been given for the amazing discoveries that have been made in how DNA stores our genetic information, how protein molecules are made up, processes that transfer materials in and out of cells, and how tiny organisms such as nematode worms are put together. But, as we shall see, this was not always the case: a very large number of Nobel Prizes have also been awarded for studies of metabolism. I should note at this point that Nobel prizes are the tip of an iceberg: most scientists beaver away, making progress that is not recognised in such a public way. But in the case of metabolism, they happen to mark a series of milestones, new developments that have shaped future thinking. Hans Krebs, perhaps the most widely known metabolic scientist, and himself a Nobel Laureate, described the situation thus: 'Nobel awards are to some measure a matter of good luck, because their number is too small to do justice to all who would merit an award . . . If I ask myself how it came about that one day I found myself in Stockholm, I have not the slightest doubt that I owe this good fortune to the circumstance that I had an outstanding teacher at the critical stage of my scientific career' (Krebs in his article 'The making of a scientist', 1967).

So, we shall spend some time looking at these pathways of metabolism, especially those concerned with fats, carbohydrates, and proteins, the three substances that provide us with energy to carry on our human lives. (We shall look a little more at this concept of 'energy' at the end of this chapter.) Ultimately, these substances release their energy for use in our muscles, our brain, heart, and other tissues by oxidation – that is, chemical reaction with oxygen. This process is related to combustion – burning – but, unlike putting a match to a candle which then burns, the process within cells involves many small chemical changes. This is critical. It enables the energy so liberated to be captured for our purposes efficiently, and also enables regulation of the processes (you can't do much to regulate a candle burning once you've started it off). It also avoids the release of a potentially destructive amount of heat within the cell. A key point that we shall meet several times – but which often seems to be overlooked by people writing about different approaches to diet – is that, ultimately, these three nutrients are broken down in the same way, and enter a 'final common pathway' for oxidation and capture of energy, the citric acid cycle, mentioned earlier. They are not independent of one another. If one substance is being oxidised, another will be spared. This is fundamental, and yet often not appreciated.

But before we get into any of these details, it will be useful to take a brief look at the history of studies of human metabolism.

How Did Our Present Views of Metabolism Evolve?

Perhaps the first scientist to begin to understand metabolism, as we now know it, was Antoine Lavoisier, the French chemist, economist, and social reformer. Lavoisier has been called the founder of modern chemistry. Since the time of the Greek philosophers, matter had been supposed to be composed of the four 'elements': Earth, Water, Air, and Fire. Lavoisier clarified the meaning of a chemical element – a substance that could not be split further into constituent parts – and he compiled a list of the elements then known. Lavoisier, like a number of scientists, especially in the UK and in France in the latter half of the eighteenth century, was interested in the composition of air, and the process of combustion. Joseph Black, a Scottish physician, and the Rev Joseph Priestley, an English minister and experimenter, had both studied the composition of air and the products of chemical reactions such as burning. These scientists distinguished what were then called different types of 'air' (using that term for what we now call a gas), such as 'fixed air', which we now call carbon dioxide, 'inflammable air' or hydrogen, and 'nitrous air' (nitrous oxide). In 1775 Priestley produced what he called 'pure air', which we now know as oxygen. He showed that a mouse could survive long periods (a couple of hours, which was longer than in other 'airs') in this gas, and tried breathing it in himself, noting that his 'breast felt particularly light and easy for some time afterwards'.

At that time, theories of burning involved a hypothetical substance 'phlogiston', which was emitted from burning matter. A substance could only continue to burn as long as the surrounding air could absorb the phlogiston emitted. Priestley did not contradict this view. He believed that his new gas, which supported combustion better than any other, must therefore initially be devoid of phlogiston, so it had a greater absorptive capacity than other gases, and accordingly he referred to it as 'dephlogisticated air'. Priestley and Lavoisier were in contact, and indeed met when Priestley visited Paris in 1774. Lavoisier had the inspiration to see that Priestley's 'dephlogisticated air' held the key to understanding combustion. Lavoisier deduced that common air was a mixture of two different components, one the newly discovered 'pure air' (oxygen), the other an inert gas that he called 'mofette', which we now call nitrogen. He showed that in combustion (the burning of a candle), the 'pure air', or as he called it, 'eminently respirable air', was consumed, and that when this was used up the combustion ended, rather than the air surrounding the candle becoming saturated with phlogiston. Lavoisier's overturning of the phlogiston theory was a major breakthrough in chemistry. In 1779, Lavoisier named this 'eminently respirable air' oxygen, from the Greek words for 'acid' and 'beget'.

Lavoisier, though, wanted to extend his research beyond the burning of candles and the oxidation of metals. Like Priestley, and Black before him, he showed that when a small animal (usually a mouse) breathed common air, 'fixed air' (carbon dioxide) was produced. He also showed that the *mofette* (nitrogen) passed into the lungs and came out unchanged. He worked with the French mathematician Pierre-Simon Laplace, to study the heat that was produced in combustion. Heat could be measured in an instrument known as a calorimeter (named from the Latin *calor* for heat, as in the calorie) – an insulated container in which a rise in temperature could be measured. They studied the heat produced by animals, devising a calorimeter in which a guinea pig could be studied for several hours. They measured the heat produced by the animal by surrounding the instrument with ice and seeing how much of the ice melted. They also measured the amount of oxygen used by the animal. In separate experiments, they showed that combustion (burning a candle) using this amount of oxygen produced a very similar amount of heat. '*La respiration*', declared Lavoisier, '*est donc une combustion*' – respiration (by which he meant the use of the air breathed in, not just the process of breathing) is a form of combustion. Lavoisier had no way of knowing what was going on inside the guinea pig's body – the requisite techniques were not available to him. But he must have realised that within the animal's lungs there was no fire, as in the burning of a candle, although the end result, in terms of heat and carbon dioxide produced, was the same.

Lavoisier extended these observations to the human body. In around 1789, he studied his assistant Armand Séguin, providing him with oxygen to breathe, and using a mask to collect the carbon dioxide produced (Figure 1.1).

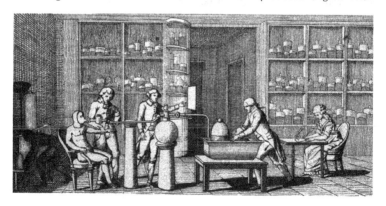

Figure 1.1 Lavoisier's experiment with his assistant Séguin.

Lavoisier was able to show that consumption of oxygen and production of carbon dioxide increased when Séguin was digesting a meal, or exercising, or subjected to a cold environment.

The tragic end to Lavoisier's experimentation came in 1794 during the Reign of Terror, when the French Revolutionary Tribunal condemned him to death on the guillotine, because he had been a tax gatherer or 'Farmer-General'. The French mathematician Lagrange remarked 'Only a moment to cut off that head, and a hundred years may not give us another like it'.

One of Lavoisier's interests had been the improvement of French agriculture. He felt it lagged behind English agriculture. He worked with the Committee of Agriculture to improve this situation, in part by increasing the number of cows and sheep raised by farmers. During the early part of the nineteenth century the raising of farm animals became an important area of scientific research. European scientists, including Justus von Liebig in Germany and Jean-Baptiste Boussingault in France, studied the role of nitrogen in crops and animals. von Liebig showed the importance of nitrogen for plant growth and speculated that nitrogen-containing substances in plants and animals were similar (we now call them proteins). Boussingault showed that plants do not use nitrogen directly from the air. Gaseous nitrogen must first be converted into other substances (starting with ammonia) from which it can become utilisable. We now know that this is done by bacteria in the soil, associated with the roots of some crops. Nitrogen is needed by animals in the form of protein (we will explore this further in later chapters), and this must arise initially from plants. (In the early twentieth century, an industrial method for converting gaseous nitrogen into ammonia, the Haber-Bosch process, was developed by the German scientists after whom it is named. This is now the major route for 'fixing' nitrogen from the air for use as a fertiliser, and ultimately for making the protein on which we depend.)

The nutritional needs of farm animals were studied at this time, essentially by measuring what the animal ate (usually something fed by the experimenters), what was excreted, and how the animal grew – or did not grow. This led to a greater understanding of the need for both protein and 'energy sources', carbohydrate and fat, for adequate growth and well-being of an animal. However, the question of what processes were going on inside the animal was still largely unanswered.

It was another French scientist who took this research forward. Claude Bernard was a French physician who studied animals – mainly dogs – in his laboratory and developed the science of the workings of the body that we now call physiology. Bernard emphasised the importance of the internal medium of the body, or 'milieu intérieur'. He believed that 'the stability of the internal environment (the milieu intérieur) is the condition for the free and independent life'. He worked on the internal processes that govern this medium, concentrating especially upon the role of the pancreas in digestion, and the liver in maintaining the correct amount of glucose (sugar) in the bloodstream – both processes that we shall explore later.

Metabolic investigations were now going to a deeper level than 'what goes in and what comes out'. By the end of the nineteenth century the emphasis had shifted further, so that now the metabolism of individual tissues (such as muscle or liver) could be investigated in the laboratory. The twentieth century saw an enormous growth in this research, with key metabolic pathways being discovered.

The German scientist Otto Warburg worked on the biochemical pathway of combustion. We saw earlier that Lavoisier had shown that fuels are used by the human body in a process with similarities to combustion. Warburg investigated just what was going on inside cells. Confusingly to the outsider, as noted before, the term 'respiration' is often used by scientists to refer to the process of using fuels by combining them with oxygen (whereas for most people, respiration refers to the act of breathing). Warburg's studies on the mechanism of respiration led in 1931 to the award of the Nobel Prize in Physiology or Medicine.

Hans Krebs, another 'giant' of metabolic research, and perhaps the only one whose name is widely known, studied medicine in Germany and worked with Warburg from 1926 to 1933, when his employment was abruptly terminated by the Nazi Party because of his Jewish ancestry. (As we shall see, this was not uncommon amongst the pioneers of cellular metabolism.) Fortunately for Krebs, and for the world of metabolism, he was offered a position in the UK, initially in Cambridge, where he continued his research into cellular respiration. He soon moved to the University of Sheffield and later, in 1954, to the University of Oxford, where he worked until his death in 1981.

Krebs is remembered especially for the discovery of two important metabolic pathways that take the form of 'cycles' – again, a concept we will explore in more detail in later chapters. The better known of these is the cycle now often known as the Krebs Cycle, more officially called the citric acid cycle, or the tricarboxylic acid cycle. We shall examine it in Chapter 5 – and see how it gets its different names. This is the common pathway by which metabolic fuels are oxidised – that is, combined with oxygen in the process analogous to combustion. As we shall explore throughout this book, this process is absolutely crucial to any understanding of what we should, or should not, eat (and whether it matters), and indeed of 'fast' or 'slow' metabolism.

The other cycle discovered by Krebs is known as the urea cycle, and takes us back to the nineteenth-century work of Boussingault and others. Animals are largely built of proteins. A characteristic of proteins is that they contain nitrogen. As these proteins are eventually broken down, this nitrogen must be disposed of. Some forms of nitrogen are quite toxic to animals, ammonia being one of these. In the urea cycle, which operates in the liver, 'unwanted' nitrogen is converted to the substance called urea, which is relatively non-toxic and is excreted in the urine. Like Warburg before him, Hans Krebs was awarded the Nobel Prize in Physiology or Medicine in 1953 for his discovery of the citric acid cycle (Figure 1.2).

Over the course of more than 150 years, then, the study of metabolism had moved from an overall view of nutrients, or fuels, being taken in, and waste products (such as carbon dioxide and urea) coming out, to detailed study of the pathways within cells that bring about these changes. To return to the

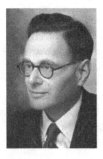

Figure 1.2 Professor Sir Hans Krebs.

analogy of economics, the science had moved from measuring GDP to exploring the myriad 'local economies' and other processes that make this up. These metabolic processes, or pathways, are what we know as 'intermediary metabolism', and we shall explore them further in the rest of this book.

Human Metabolism in a Wider Context

We shall be exploring the means by which we, humans, derive energy from our foodstuffs. It's useful at the outset just to think about where this energy came from. We eat plant and animal tissues. All the energy 'stored' in these comes originally from the sun. Plant cells use the energy in sunlight to make sugars through a process called photosynthesis. These sugars are the starting point for making starches and also fats. As noted above, soil bacteria can use nitrogen from the atmosphere and incorporate it into organic compounds, which are taken up by plants, which we eat in turn. Even the meat-eaters amongst us are dependent upon these plant sources: if you eat beef, for instance, the cow will have derived its bodily materials by eating plants – no animal has the ability to capture and use the energy of sunlight, nor to incorporate nitrogen from the air into its bodily materials. Ultimately, then, when I pedal my bicycle up the hill that connects our residential area to the centre of Oxford, I am using energy derived from sunlight – my bicycle is (indirectly) solar powered!

In general, as molecules get bigger, they store more energy. Life centres on molecules built of carbon (C) atoms. During photosynthesis, plants use carbon dioxide (CO_2) from the air and, with energy from sunlight, convert this into sugars. A typical sugar molecule, such as glucose, has six atoms of carbon ($C_6H_{12}O_6$, meaning its molecules each contain six atoms of carbon, 12 of hydrogen and six of oxygen). Fats are mostly built of units called fatty acids (more detail in the next chapter). A common fatty acid, palmitic acid, has 16 carbon atoms in each molecule. The process of making more complex molecules from simpler ones is called anabolism.

Breaking down of complex molecules is called catabolism. As these complex molecules are broken down by combination with oxygen, the process of

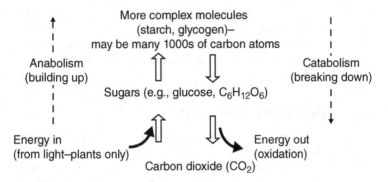

Figure 1.3 Anabolism and catabolism. This is shown for sugars, but sugars can be converted into fats and amino acids and similar pathways operate. We could say that 'metabolism' is the sum of anabolism and catabolism.

oxidation, the carbon atoms are split apart, combined with oxygen, and energy is liberated. On complete combustion of glucose, just carbon dioxide and water remain, as follows:

One molecule of glucose + six molecules of oxygen → six molecules each of carbon dioxide and water;

or, in short,

$$C_6H_{12}O_6 + 6O_2 \rightarrow 6CO_2 + 6H_2O, \quad \textit{plus energy liberated}.$$

When we begin, later, to look at the cellular pathways by which this is brought about, the concept of breaking down larger molecules to make smaller ones, with release of energy, will be central to our thinking. It is illustrated in Figure 1.3.

What Is Metabolism? Conclusion

So we see that metabolism underlies all processes that keep us alive: making the components of our cells, providing energy in a continuous way for living and working, and disposing of bodily components that are no longer needed. This must involve energy stores where excess fuel can be sequestered, to be called upon when needed. We have also seen that, in order to keep metabolism doing what it needs to at any one time, a system of internal communication is needed. We shall explore each of these themes in the next few chapters.

2 Metabolic Fuels

Humans, like the Cordless Vacuum Cleaner, Have Fuel Stores

It's time to clean the carpets. I plug in the vacuum cleaner and switch on at the socket. Then I switch the machine on and start work. Considerable energy is needed creating and maintaining suction and beating the carpet at the same time. Whatever energy I need the machine to use, luckily comes straight down the cable at just the right time. If I turn on 'boost', the rate at which electrical power comes down the cable increases to match. Great job done. Now I turn the machine off and unplug it, and even if I were to try to turn it on, it won't respond.

My neighbours are more up to date with household appliances and have a cordless vacuum cleaner. Now they are independent of the power supply. Their vacuum cleaner works even though not connected to the mains electricity. And when it is at rest, not working, they connect it to the mains to take in energy. So there is no relationship in time between taking in energy and expending it. It is not like my vacuum cleaner: as mine expends energy sucking in dust, that energy is being supplied through a cord as it is used. The key difference, of course, is that my neighbours' machine has a means of storing fuel – namely a battery. It's rather like our car, which also happens to be battery powered. We charge the car when it's stationary, but discharge it when we drive. The car has a fuel store – the battery – and also a means of regulating the flow of energy to the engine, the accelerator pedal.

After all that housework, I feel like a brisk walk in the countryside. That means expending some energy – I will want to climb that hill, I am walking against the wind, and my boots use energy through friction with the ground. I might feel as though I want to drink an energy drink as I go – but I don't need to. I had a good breakfast a couple of hours ago, before the housework. I think I'll manage a couple of hills, then stop for my sandwiches. Whilst I am sitting eating them, of course, I am expending very little energy, but taking in energy rather fast. This is rather similar to the cordless vacuum cleaner or the motor car – I can take in fuel at intervals, then I can use the energy contained in it whilst no further fuel is going in via my mouth. So, of course, we deduce that humans are 'cordless': we must have a fuel tank.

Actually, humans are much more complex than these machines. Cars have just one type of fuel (two for hybrids), and they have an intelligent being who will intervene to regulate the supply of fuel to the engine. The human body, in contrast, has a variety of fuels available (although under many circumstances two, carbohydrate and fat, predominate), and a number of different engines – that is, tissues requiring fuel, such as the muscles, the heart, the lungs, and the brain – each of which will have its own particular requirements for the fuel mix at different times. And what's more, who is controlling the throttle? Nobody, at least not consciously. This is all part of the wonder of how human metabolism is regulated.

We have stores of both carbohydrates and fats. We also have a lot of protein: I shall explain later why it is different. Most people have an idea of the difference between carbohydrates and fats in a culinary sense. Carbohydrates are the basis of starchy foods, cereals and other staples: flour, bread, pasta, rice, cassava, millet and others. Fats, in contrast, are oily or greasy: animal fats, vegetable oils, and other types of oil such as fish oil. The difference between carbohydrates and fats is fundamental to understanding their role in metabolism.

Carbohydrates: The Bread of Metabolism

Much of what we are made of consists of 'polymers', a term that is familiar to most people when we talk about plastics, but not necessarily in relation to the body. A polymer is a substance whose molecules are made up of many smaller molecules, or monomers – usually, but not always, identical – joined together. Starchy substances are exactly that. The building blocks are called sugars, and again these are familiar in the kitchen: for instance, glucose ('grape sugar') and fructose ('fruit sugar'). (The names were given in the early nineteenth century, when there was agreement that sugar names would end in '-ose'.) Table sugar is called sucrose, and its molecules consist of a glucose molecule joined to one of fructose – hence it is called a disaccharide ('two sugars'). These molecules can join together in long strings – very long, with maybe tens of thousands of sugar molecules in one molecule of what we would now call a polysaccharide. And that is exactly what starch is – and also cellulose, which makes up plant cell walls and is used to make paper. They are polymers – long strings – of glucose molecules joined together. The crucial difference from fats is that sugars will dissolve readily in water – rather obvious when we think of a cup of coffee with sugar added, and quite unlike what would happen were we by accident to add a teaspoon of olive oil instead.

The ability of sugars to dissolve freely in water gives them a very special role in metabolism – especially the sugar glucose, which is the main sugar in our bodies. It means it can travel freely through the bloodstream, from one organ to another, without forming clumps that would cause problems.

And, just as plants have developed the ability to join many, many sugar units together to make starch for storage, so have animals. Animal starch is called glycogen, and chemically its structure is very similar to plant starch.

Figure 2.1 shows models of a glucose molecule and a molecule of glycogen.

Anyone who cooks will know that starch – in the form of flour – will also mix with water, although, as my own attempts at making white sauces regularly demonstrate, not actually dissolving as readily as sugar might. My wife and I have started buying fresh pasta from Danilo, an ebullient Sicilian who sells the produce of southern Italy at our local market in Oxford. We have just cooked some of Danilo's *paccheri* – 'Fresh pasta from durum wheat semolina'. We went for the al dente feel, but still, the pasta was a lot softer after cooking than before – but it hadn't actually dissolved. Had we continued cooking, no doubt it would have got softer and softer and eventually disintegrated – and dissolved to some extent. It was my job to drain the pasta, which I did by pouring it into a colander. After eating, we cleared up. The colander looked clean and I thought I might be able to put it away – but actually it was very slimy. That was the dissolved starch. Had I needed to stiffen up my shirt before work tomorrow, this would have been the ideal stuff to do it. Indeed, that's the origin of the term 'starch': the water left over after cooking

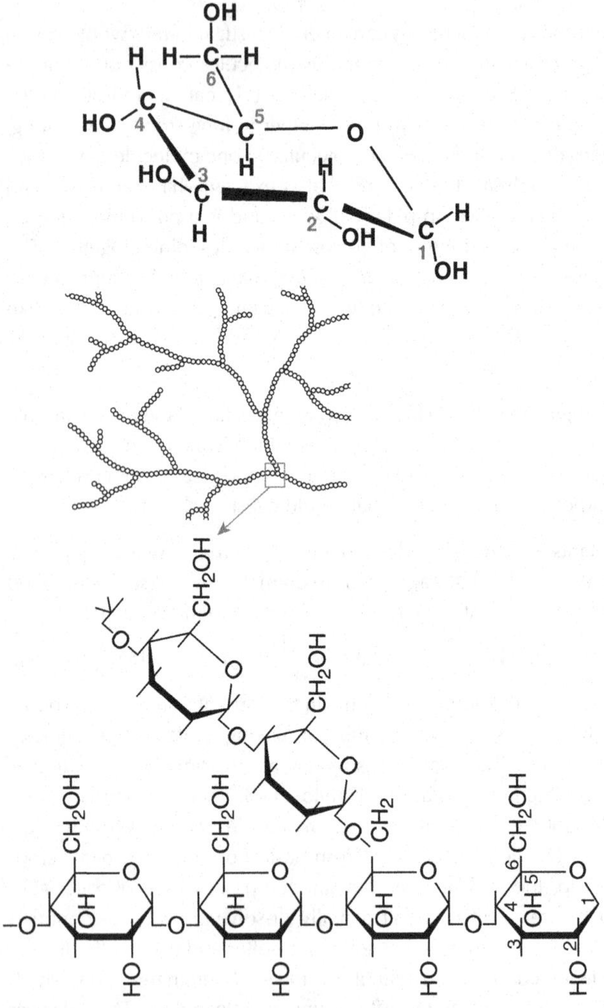

Figure 2.1   Model of a glucose molecule, and how glycogen is made up.
Each molecule of glucose has six carbon atoms (C), to which are attached oxygen (O)
and hydrogen (H) atoms. The molecule tends to adopt the shape shown, which is known
as the 'chair' configuration.
The sketch below shows how glucose molecules can join together in branching chains
to make the large polymer called glycogen ('animal starch') – the form in which we
store carbohydrate.

something starchy, which has enough of the carbohydrate material in solution that when applied to fabric and ironed in, it will cause the fabric to remain stiff ('starched'). Even cellulose, which is a tough substance derived from plant cell walls, will mix to some extent with water, making a sort of paste – such as wallpaper paste. Glycogen is the same – it mixes with water, indeed in our cells is always intimately connected with water. That will be important when we consider glycogen as an energy source.

Fats: The Butter of Metabolism

Not all substances dissolve readily in, or mix easily with, water.

Fat is a very general term – it derives from the Old English word for 'to cram' or 'stuff'. Another term commonly used in science is 'lipid', which is of twentieth-century origin from the Greek *lipos* for fat. The definition of fats or lipids is that they are unable to dissolve in water, although they will dissolve in stronger solvents such as petroleum or chloroform. A very large number of materials fall into this category including waxes, oils, and solid fats. However, to bring us back to human metabolism, we will consider two groups of fats.

Cholesterol is a type of fat called a steroid. As we all know, it is present in the bloodstream and has a role in the development of heart disease. It is there to help transport other lipids around the bloodstream, it is a constituent of cell membranes, and it is also a precursor for some hormones (such as cortisol). But cholesterol does not play a role in 'energy metabolism' (by which I mean a consideration of those materials we might consider fuels for the body), so we will not consider it further here.

We shall spend much more time looking at fats that are built from a smaller unit called the fatty acid. Why fatty acid? These substances are fatty, and only very slightly soluble in water: but if we test that water, we find it is acidic. They are weak acids though, and not going to burn through your intestines like sulphuric acid might. Why are fatty acids soluble in water to any extent, when I said that in general fats don't dissolve in water? Because of the very interesting structure of their molecules. These are mainly water-insoluble (fatty), but have one water-soluble end (the acid end). The technical term for a material that mixes well with water is hydrophilic (literally meaning 'water-friendly'), whereas the opposite is hydrophobic ('water-fearing'). Shortly we shall see that this property of fatty acids has made them a valuable commodity in the house – and not just as a fuel for our cells. They make up soap.

There are different types of fatty acid, commonly known as saturated and unsaturated. For our purposes here, discussing fuel stores, they are essentially the same. 'Saturation' is a chemical term, meaning that the molecule is 'saturated' (or completed) with hydrogen. Fatty acid molecules consist of chains of carbon atoms, most commonly 16 or 18 carbon atoms, in a line, one joined to the next. If all 'spare' chemical bonds are occupied by hydrogen atoms, then the molecule is 'saturated' and adopts a fairly straight shape. If, on the other hand, one pair of carbon atoms lacks these hydrogen atoms, the adjacent carbon atoms join together in a different way (usually called a 'double bond') and this introduces a bend, or kink, into the molecule. You can see this in Figure 2.2.

Fatty acids can join, through their acid group, to another molecule. It's a common bond between molecules in biology – an acid joins to something that belongs to the chemical group of alcohols. It is called an ester link. In the case of fatty acids in the body, this link is most commonly with a compound called glycerol. Glycerol, also called glycerine, is a common constituent of skin creams. Skin is rich in glycerol, which helps keep it moist – hence, it is

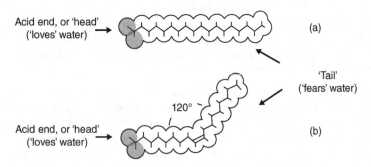

Figure 2.2 Models of molecules of two different fatty acids: (a) palmitic acid, the most common saturated fatty acid (it has 16 carbon atoms), and (b) oleic acid, the most common unsaturated fatty acid, with 18 carbon atoms and one 'double bond', introducing a kink into the molecule. The solid black line in the middle represents a chain of carbon atoms, with hydrogen atoms at each joint.

added to moisturising creams. You will see that much of this concerns household commodities.

Glycerol molecules are small (in biological terms) – they have three carbon atoms, and each of these has an 'alcohol' group (it is called a trihydric alcohol). It is, therefore, related chemically to ethanol – the alcohol in alcoholic drinks – but doesn't have the same effects. Three fatty acid molecules can then join with ester links to one of glycerol. The resulting compound is called a triacylglycerol ('acyl' meaning deriving from a fatty acid) or, especially in older literature, a triglyceride. A model of a molecule of a triacylglycerol is shown in Figure 2.3. Maybe the term triacylglycerol conjures up a chemistry laboratory. But it shouldn't: this is what we commonly call fat in the kitchen. Animal fats, vegetable oils, fish oil: all triacylglycerols. And, indeed, human fat – that stuff many of us feel we have too much of – is made of triacylglycerols.

Different fats in the kitchen clearly differ in their appearance. Animal fats, like lard or dairy fat in butter, and a few vegetable fats, such as palm oil, are relatively solid. Vegetable oils, on the other hand, are more liquid. The harder fats have mostly saturated fatty acids (completed with hydrogen). Because their molecules are relatively straight, they can line up and pack together closely. This makes them solid. Vegetable oils, on the other hand, contain

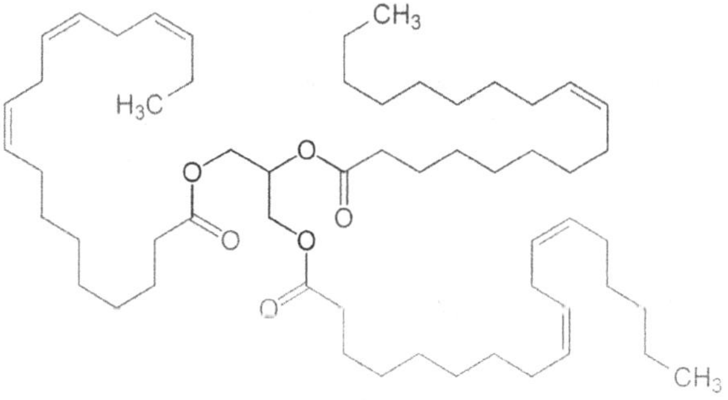

Figure 2.3 Model of the structure of a molecule of a triacylglycerol (e.g. it might be a vegetable oil in the kitchen). The black structure in the centre is the glycerol molecule: the outer grey structures are three different unsaturated fatty acids. (Saturated fatty acids would have a straighter conformation, as you can see in Figure 2.2).

unsaturated fatty acids, and their bent shapes (as in Figure 2.3) mean that they form looser collections, and tend to be liquid. Oleic acid, shown in Figure 2.2, has one 'double bond' and is called 'monounsaturated'. It is a major component of the triacylglycerols making up olive oil (hence the name, from the Latin *oleum*, oil). Other fatty acids have more 'double bonds' and more kinks, and are even more liquid – they are described as polyunsaturated. Olive oil will solidify in a refrigerator, but sunflower oil, for instance, is polyunsaturated, and will remain liquid even in the cold.

Carbohydrates and Fats as Fuel Stores

We need to consider how much energy is stored in carbohydrates and fats. In case it's useful, Box 2.1 is a little primer on measurements of energy.

Carbohydrates are stored as glycogen, within the cells of many of our tissues. Some tissues, including the brain, have a small amount of glycogen, but most of our glycogen is stored in our muscles and liver. Glycogen is a source of the

Box 2.1 Units of energy balance.

Traditionally, energy in foodstuffs was measured in units based on the calorie. One calorie is the energy needed to heat 1 gram (g) of water by 1 centigrade degree (C°). It is a tiny amount. In nutrition, it became traditional to use kilocalories (kcal), where 1 kcal = 1 000 calories. Some nutritionists adopted the practice of calling 1 kcal one Calorie (with a capital C). This is potentially very confusing and best avoided! But you may see these units in diet books.

Nowadays, most scientists use a system of measures based on metres, kilograms, and seconds. In this system, energy is defined on the basis of force and distance, where force is itself based on mass and acceleration. The unit of energy in this system is the joule, abbreviated J. One calorie is equal to 4.18 J. Again, like the calorie, the joule is a tiny amount of energy, and for nutritional purposes it's most useful to work in kilojoules (kJ) or megajoules (MJ), where

1 kJ = 1 000 J (about 0.24 kcal)
1 MJ = 1 000 kJ = 1 000,000 J (about 240 kcal)

Because many people still think in kcal, I will always give the conversion from joules (J) to calories.

sugar glucose, which is an important metabolic fuel. As a round figure, we might have a few hundred grams stored in our muscles, and about 100 g in our liver – maybe 500 g in all. We will see later that there is a difference between muscle and liver stores, though: the main purpose of the glycogen in muscles is to provide fuel for those muscles, whereas the liver stores glycogen in order to supply the rest of the body with glucose.

The human brain needs glucose. Only under some extreme circumstances will it use other fuels. Our brains need around 100–120 g of glucose each day. It is surely no coincidence that this is almost exactly the amount stored in the liver. Our liver glycogen provides a ready source of energy for the brain should we go for 24 hours without eating. (Beyond that, very interesting changes take place to enable us to survive fasting – of which more later.)

We understand the role of the liver glycogen store because of some rather heroic experiments conducted in Sweden in the 1970s. Two Swedish researchers (Lars Nilsson and Eric Hultman in Stockholm) recruited healthy (and brave) volunteers to study the amount of glycogen in the liver. Taking a liver biopsy (a small sample of the liver, taken with a long, fine needle inserted into the abdomen) is a fairly serious procedure. The volunteers had liver samples taken at the beginning, then they began to starve. After 24 hours without food, there was virtually no glycogen left in the liver. Some volunteers then starved entirely for 10 days. And the glycogen remained almost absent until the volunteers were fed again on day 11, when the amount of glycogen shot quickly back to pre-starvation levels. Glycogen in the liver is a 24-hour reserve, essentially to keep our brains going.

One gram of glucose, when combined with oxygen, releases energy: around 17 kJ (4 kcal). So, 100 g of glycogen in the liver represents around 1 700 kJ (1.7 MJ – or 400 kcal). If we add in the muscle store, say 500 g in all, that represents 8 500 kcal (8.5 MJ – or 2 030 kcal) – approaching one day's-worth of energy if it were all used.

So what fuel were the starving volunteers using after their liver glycogen store was depleted? The answer is, of course, fat, drawn from their fat stores. In terms of energy stored, we all of us have much more in the form of fat than we do carbohydrate. Clearly the amount of fat stored varies enormously from one person to another. So where to start?

My colleague Professor Fredrik Karpe maintains a database of adult people randomly recruited from the local Oxfordshire population, called the Oxford BioBank (OBB). Fredrik has kindly sent me data on 1 500 of these people, men and women. They have all had a thorough investigation in the laboratory, which includes measurement of their fat mass – the amount of fat in the body. The average figure is 25 kilograms (kg) so let's work with this. (Out of interest, the lowest fat mass amongst this group was 6 kg, the greatest 68 kg. This just shows how it varies from person to person.)

When fat is combined with oxygen, energy is released, about 37 kJ/g (9 kcal/g). Multiplying up, 25 kg fat would provide around 945 000 kJ, or 945 MJ (226 000 kcal). As we shall see in more detail later, the human body needs around 10 MJ per day (2 500 kcal in round figures) for normal living (again a ball-park figure), so we have enough energy for around 90 days stored as fat. Again, I stress that this may be much less – or much more – depending on the individual.

We see immediately that much more energy is stored as fat than as carbohydrate in the human body. That applies even to thin people.

Carbohydrates versus Fats as Fuel Stores

Why have we evolved to store most of our energy in the form of fat rather than carbohydrate? The answer will jump out at you from Figure 2.4.

As we have just seen, for a given weight, fat stores considerably more energy than carbohydrate. A carbohydrate like starch, or a sugar like glucose, liberates about 17 kJ/g (4 kcal/g) on combustion. But, by its very nature, carbohydrate does not exist in the body in a dry form; it is always associated with water. Glycogen is stored with about three times its own weight of water. This means that every 17 kJ stored will add about 4 g in weight. We see that 100 g, as stored in the body with water, will provide about 415 kJ (100 kcal).

Fat, on the other hand, in the form of triacylglycerol, is stored almost entirely without water. It is stored mostly in specialised 'fat cells', called adipocytes. These cells contain very little other than a droplet of fat: maybe 10% of their weight will be cell water, nucleus, and other components. Triacylglycerols liberate about 37 kJ/g (9 kcal/g) when combusted. If we reduce this by 10% to allow for the water, then 100 g of fat tissue will store about 3 330 kJ, or 3.3 MJ

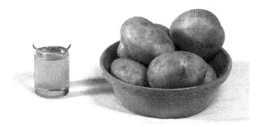

Figure 2.4 Fat and carbohydrate as energy stores. The picture shows 90 g of olive oil and 1.05 kg of raw potatoes. Each provides 3.3 megajoules (MJ) of energy (800 kcal). Raw potatoes contain a similar amount of water to our glycogen stores – about three times the weight of carbohydrate.

[about 790 kcal/100 g]: something like eight times as much as hydrated glycogen. Carrying our energy mainly as fat rather than as carbohydrate means that we can walk around all day carrying a sufficient energy store, in case we face a considerable period without eating.

Storing and Mobilising Our Reserves: Just like Making Soap!

A major theme in this book will be metabolic pathways – a term we shall explore in the next chapter – for directing spare nutrients into our energy stores, and for getting them out of those stores when we require them. Here's a quick overview.

When we eat starchy foods, the starch is broken down in our small intestine to release the sugars of which it is made up. If we eat sugary foods, that step is unnecessary. Then the sugars – mainly glucose in most circumstances – can be taken up, through the cells that line the small intestine, into the blood. The bloodstream is a major motorway (or freeway): substances can travel from one part of the body to another, from one tissue to another. In the case of sugars, this is easy – the sugar is dissolved in the watery part of the blood, the plasma. As blood reaches each organ or tissue, it finds itself directed into smaller and smaller side-streets, the capillaries. Just as a parcel might be sent out from a central delivery point, and makes its way along major roads, then later along smaller side-streets, to reach a given destination, so it is with substances carried in the bloodstream.

'Ah', you may say, 'but the glucose molecules don't carry an address label. How do they know where to knock on the door and go in?'

This is all part of the beauty of metabolism, and we will explore the answer more as we go along. But here's a start. Much of the glucose we eat will make its way to the liver. That's partly because the layout of our circulatory system has evolved to give sugars absorbed from the intestine direct access to the liver. The blood vessels that leave the small intestine, carrying the dissolved nutrients, merge and make their way directly to the liver through a large vessel called the hepatic portal vein (hepatic meaning to do with the liver). When a glucose molecule passes through a capillary in the liver, it may find itself drawn down a gradient of concentration towards some holes in a liver cell's membrane which are made by specific proteins called glucose transporters: their structure is such that glucose molecules, but nothing else, can pass through. The glucose molecule is drawn into the cell because, inside the liver cell, changes have happened that mean the cell's machinery is ready to process it along a metabolic pathway – that we are just about to explore. And how did the liver cell know to expect, and be ready to process, the glucose molecule? The answer is that it is forewarned of the glucose molecule's arrival! That is the marvel of metabolic communication systems, which we shall discuss in Chapter 4.

So, glucose arrives in the liver, and within the liver cells metabolic pathways are primed to stick glucose molecules together in chains to make the starch-like storage molecules that we call glycogen. Hence we build up our glycogen store, that will have been depleted as we dipped into it before the meal. But, looking ahead a little, after the meal has gone down, we will need to draw again upon that glycogen store. So, then a pathway comes into action that breaks glucose molecules, one by one, off the glycogen molecules, and these glucose molecules can be released from the liver cells into the bloodstream and travel to places that are now calling out for them – the brain, for instance. These pathways we would broadly characterise as glucose storage, after a meal, and glucose (or glycogen) mobilisation, between meals.

And just the same will happen with fat – although, because fat molecules are not soluble in water, the process is a little more complex. Fat that we eat, made of triacylglycerols, is digested in the small intestine. Much of it is broken down to release the fatty acids. These fatty acids, and some partially broken-down triacylglycerol molecules, will enter the cells lining the small intestine.

Here, the fatty acids are recombined with the glycerol 'backbone' to make triacylglycerol molecules.

But here's the complication. These triacylglycerol molecules are not soluble in the blood. Indeed, that's the very reason, as we have seen, that they are so ideal as a long-term store of energy. They can only enter the bloodstream by coming together in minute (sub-microscopic) droplets which are held together with other fats and specific proteins. These droplets, as I will call them (the term 'particles' is often used in scientific work), are very, very similar to the fat droplets that give milk its white colour. Fat droplets in milk scatter the light that passes through to make milk opaque, and in just the same way, these particles will make the blood plasma cloudy (Figure 2.5).

These fatty droplets don't follow the same path as the glucose. They are taken up from the intestinal cells into little vessels that are part of the lymphatic system. The lymphatic system consists of a series of vessels whose main role is

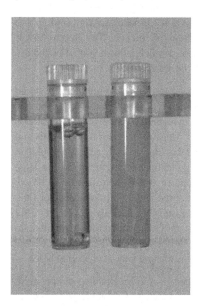

Figure 2.5 Blood plasma (blood with the red blood cells removed): on the left, taken after fasting overnight; on the right, taken a few hours after a fatty meal. The plasma has turned cloudy, like milk, because of the presence of fat that came from the meal.

to drain excess fluid from tissues. It also has a role in immunity. These little lymph vessels that drain the small intestine are called lacteals – the term coming from the Latin word *lac*, for milk, because they look milky after a fatty meal. They merge into a larger lymph vessel that travels up the back of the abdomen and chest and discharges its milky contents into the bloodstream near the neck. Nobody can really explain why this is so.

So now we have milky droplets containing fat (triacylglycerol) that we have eaten, going round the bloodstream. When they come into the capillaries of certain tissues, they will meet an enzyme, attached to the walls of the capillaries, that breaks down the triacylglycerol molecules yet again, releasing fatty acids, that enter the adjacent cells. (Some might simply diffuse through the membrane, which is itself made of fatty molecules, but some will find proteins that make fatty acid-shaped holes for them – fatty acid transporters.)

After a meal much of this fat will be directed to our adipose tissue, where we store fat (in fat cells, or adipocytes). Here, as you might already guess, the fatty acids are combined yet again with glycerol to make triacylglycerol which then joins the pool of triacylglycerol already in the cell. (The glycerol in this case is made from glucose.) So this is the parallel pathway to that of glucose making glycogen – it is the pathway of fat storage.

Just as with carbohydrates, when we need to use this stored fuel, the stored molecules, triacylglycerols, are broken down to release fatty acids. And it is these fatty acids that now become the 'dynamic currency' of fat metabolism, like sugars in the case of carbohydrates. They are released from fat cells into the bloodstream. But I have already said that they are only a tiny bit soluble in the blood plasma. They get carried round by hitching a lift on the large molecules of the protein called albumin, of which there is a lot in blood. They bind loosely to albumin, perhaps three fatty acid molecules per molecule of albumin: when they reach a tissue that is ready to use them (for instance, muscles, if we are exercising), they will unhitch from the albumin and enter the muscle cells – again, maybe some will diffuse into the cell, but others will enter through specific proteins making fatty-acid-shaped holes.

You will see that, in fat metabolism, there is a lot of shuttling of fatty acids between triacylglycerol molecules and 'unattached' fatty acids. (In the UK we tend to call these non-esterified fatty acids, NEFA, whereas in American literature free fatty acids, FFA, is commonly used.)

Here again there's a relationship with domestic affairs. The process of breaking down triacylglycerols to make fatty acids is chemically exactly the same as making soap from vegetable or animal fats. In the human body, this conversion is brought about by enzymes (proteins that facilitate chemical reactions – more in the next chapter on enzymes). In soap-making it is brought about by a strong alkali, usually sodium hydroxide (caustic soda). Soap consists of fatty acids in the form of their sodium salts. You will remember that triacylglycerol molecules also contain glycerol. Glycerol can also be part of soap because, as I mentioned earlier, it is good for moisturising the skin.

But there is a difference. No soap-maker has ever managed to recombine the fatty acids back into triacylglycerols (or probably even tried to); and yet, this happens all the time in human metabolism – as we have already seen.

But why soap? What do fatty acids have to do with washing your hands? This ability comes about because of their dual nature. Most dirt that will not wash off readily in water is oil-based or greasy. Fatty acids, especially in the form of sodium salts (when the properties of the 'water-friendly' end are especially pronounced), can bridge the gap between grease and water. The water-fearing (oil-friendly) tails of the fatty acids will dip into the dirt, and the water-friendly ends will be exposed to the water, enabling sub-microscopic droplets of fat to be washed off, surrounded by fatty acids. (Something very similar happens when fats are transported round the body.)

Proteins

You may be wondering why we have got so far without discussing the third major component of the foods we eat – proteins. And not just of foods we eat – also a major component of the body. Many tissues are made up of, firstly, water, and secondly, protein. Muscles, for example, are (approximately) 70% water, 25% protein, and 5% other things (e.g. fat, glycogen) by weight; liver is similar. A typical person holds about 10–15 kg of protein in his or her tissues, which may be greater than the amount of fat (in a thin person), and an order of magnitude more than our carbohydrate store.

Just as we have seen for carbohydrates and fats, proteins are polymers made up from many smaller units. These units are the amino acids. An amino acid is a compound whose molecules have two characteristic components: a group that contains a nitrogen atom, called the amino group ($-NH_2$), and an acid group (−COOH): hence their name. The various amino acids (there are 20 that make up most proteins) differ in the other things attached, mainly chains or rings of carbon atoms of various lengths, from no additional carbon atoms (the amino acid called glycine), up to nine in the amino acid tryptophan. They join together in strings, one amino acid's amino group linking to another's acid group. The link is called a peptide bond. A string of up to about 10 amino acids is called a peptide, beyond that the string is called a polypeptide or a protein. The largest protein in the human body is called titin, an elastic component of muscles, with around 30 000 amino acids, in a strictly defined order. Figure 2.6 shows some amino acids, and how they link together to form proteins. Box 2.2 tells you a little about chemical structures, with which you may not be familiar, and how they will be used in this book.

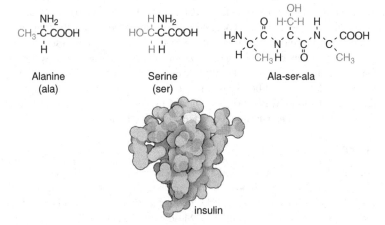

Figure 2.6 Models of two amino acids, a small peptide, and a representation of the structure of a protein (the hormone insulin).
Alanine (ala) and serine (ser) are two common amino acids. Their common components are shown in black: their specific parts are in grey. Amino acids link together through peptide bonds. Here the hypothetical tripeptide ala-ser-ala is shown. Also shown is a representation of the three-dimensional structure of a protein, the hormone insulin (discussed in Chapter 4), which has 51 amino acids joined sequentially in a specific order, giving it its shape and function. (Many proteins have several hundred or even thousands of amino acids.)

Box 2.2. A note on chemical structures.

In the course of our journey through metabolism we will meet a few chemical formulae, in different forms. When scientists depict a glucose molecule as $C_6H_{12}O_6$, this is called the molecular formula, and tells us the composition of each molecule in terms of atoms (six carbon atoms, 12 of hydrogen, and six of oxygen in this case). The molecular formula tells you nothing about how the atoms are linked together. That needs a structural formula, like the amino acids shown in Figure 2.6. But these molecules also have three-dimensional form, as shown for glucose in Figure 2.1. Sometimes a simplified, linear structural formula is used: alanine (Figure 2.6) would be shown as CH_3CHNH_2COOH.

The molecular and structural formulae in this book are over-simplified. The acid group, $-COOH$, is usually present in 'dissociated' form: the hydrogen separates as a positively charged ion, leaving a negative ion behind: $-COO^-$ and H^+. That's what makes it an acid. Similarly, basic (alkaline) groups like the amino group, $-NH_2$, will tend to be associated with a hydrogen ion, so they become $-NH_3^+$. I haven't shown that, for simplicity. When lactic acid, for instance, dissociates we have:

| $CH_3CHOHCOOH$ | $\leftrightarrow$ | $CH_3CHOHCOO^-$ | $+$ | H^+ |
| Lactic acid (undissociated) | | Lactate ion | | Hydrogen ion |

This explains why you often see 'lactic acid' referred to as 'lactate'. (It is almost entirely dissociated in our bodies.) Think of them as the same thing.

It's definitely not necessary to remember the formulae: the main thing to bear in mind is simply how many carbon atoms are in the molecules of each compound we meet.

The key feature of a protein is that it consists of a string of amino acids in a defined order and number. It is this sequence of amino acids in each protein that is encoded in our genes, our DNA. Our DNA prescribes the number and order of amino acids in each of our proteins. We have something like 25 000 genes coding for proteins, meaning that a complement of a few tens of thousands of different proteins is enough to determine that I shall be me, and not you, or a chimpanzee, or even a daisy. Proteins are quite remarkable in the range of functions that they may carry out. They can do this because each type of amino acid has particular chemical properties, giving the complete protein molecule a specific shape and properties. We shall shortly meet proteins that bring about chemical reactions, called enzymes, and also proteins that sit in the membranes of cells and allow smaller molecules through (such as the glucose transporters), or receive messages from hormones in the blood.

When we eat protein, it is digested in the stomach and small intestine, and, just like sugars and fats, the smaller sub-units, amino acids, are taken up into the bloodstream through the intestinal wall. (Some dipeptides, i.e. two amino acids joined, can also be taken up.) Like glucose, amino acids are carried straight to the liver, and some will enter liver cells; some will go through the liver into the general bloodstream, and hence reach other tissues.

So, our tissues are made of proteins, and nearly all cells in the human body can use amino acids – delivered in the bloodstream – to make new proteins, but also break down proteins to release amino acids; there is always a turnover of proteins, presumably so that as they age and are perhaps damaged in cells, they are replaced with new ones.

Amino acids, just like glucose and fatty acids, can be broken down to liberate energy. A general figure would be that amino acids on combustion liberate around 17 kJ/g, like carbohydrates (4 kcal/g). A ballpark figure for protein content of an adult human might be 12.5 kg, so this represents around 210 000 kJ or 210 MJ (51 000 kcal) – apparently enough to provide for 3 weeks or so of our energy needs. So, why didn't I include protein in the list of fuel stores that enable me to climb hills without drinking my energy drink as I go?

The answer is contained in the previous sections. Glycogen in liver and muscle cells has but one function: it is there to be broken down, to release glucose when needed. Fat in our fat cells is the same: in itself it does nothing, it is there purely to liberate its fatty acids when they are needed. But this is not so with proteins. Every molecule of protein in our bodies has a function. There is no specific storage form of protein. So, if we were to use proteins for energy, we would be depleting the body of some function. In fact, as we will see later, the human body is remarkably tenacious in holding onto its proteins, even in complete starvation: carbohydrates and, especially, fats will be used in preference. Only when the fat stores have really gone will the body dip into its protein reserve for energy, and that is not compatible for long with life.

Fuel Stores and Metabolism

At the end of Chapter 1, we looked at an overview of how energy from sunlight allows plants to use carbon dioxide from the atmosphere to build up more complex molecules: initially sugars such as glucose, but from these can be formed fats and (with some input from other organisms) amino acids. These 'monomers' can in turn be combined to make more complex molecules, the process of 'anabolism' (illustrated in Figure 1.3). The opposite process, breaking them down and releasing energy (ultimately, by combination with oxygen – oxidation) is called 'catabolism'. These terms are also used at a whole-body level. When someone is growing, we describe that as anabolism; if someone is ill, for instance, and losing tissues, we say they are in a catabolic state.

So, we have met, at least in outline, some of the key pathways of metabolism. Before we go much further, we need to look in more detail at what is meant by a metabolic pathway, and how the flow of substances along a metabolic pathway can be regulated.

3 Metabolic Pathways

The Concept of Metabolic Pathways

In Chapter 1, I slipped into using the term 'metabolic pathway' without much explanation. Metabolic pathways are the roadmap of metabolism. If we wish to understand human metabolism, and how it relates to our daily lives, we will need an understanding of this term; so in this chapter I shall offer a quick guide, and show how our views have changed over the years.

Most of the metabolic pathways that underlie the use of nutrients and their utilisation as fuels, or conversion into the substance of the body, had been at least outlined by the 1950s. This came about through the work of the cellular biochemists whom we met in Chapter 1. Since that time, further details of some pathways have been elucidated, but the main increase in knowledge has been in the area of 'regulation'. We can envisage materials following a pathway (like water flowing through a pipe); but, as we saw in the previous chapter, this flow is not constant in time, but can be switched on or off, or regulated to be less or more. This understanding has largely come about through detailed studies of the enzymes that make metabolism happen, as we shall see shortly. More recently, in the past decade or so, new methods have been used to look at 'fingerprints' of metabolic products in cells or tissues, or even blood or urine samples. These techniques have given us new insights into how metabolic pathways inter-relate, and have shown the importance of some key compounds that are at the intersection of different metabolic pathways.

Metabolic Pathways Typically Involve Many Small Steps

When we eat foods containing carbohydrate ('starchy foods'), much of the starch is converted in the intestine to the sugar called glucose and enters the bloodstream. From here different tissues can extract the glucose: for instance, muscles may use this glucose to produce the force needed for physical work. A major metabolic pathway is the route by which glucose within a cell is fully 'combusted': broken down, combined with oxygen, O_2, producing just carbon dioxide, CO_2, and water, H_2O (plus energy released). This process is called oxidation. Glucose will burn in a flame, but clearly this is not what happens in our cells. Instead, there is a series of small chemical changes, which sequentially prepare the molecules of glucose for their breakdown, and then break them apart, little by little. It may be likened to one of those puzzles in which one word must be transformed into another by changing just one letter at a time:

Dog → cog → cot → cat

More appropriately, the word is shortened, or the molecule broken down, in some of the steps:

Book → took → too (+k) → to (+o)

We don't need to know all the steps in the breakdown of glucose, but this pathway consists of two parts. First, the glucose molecule is effectively broken in half, then each half may, or may not, enter the citric acid (Krebs) cycle, mentioned in Chapter 1, for final conversion to CO_2. A little chemical nomenclature here may help to explain, but it's not essential. The molecule of glucose (see Figure 2.1) has six carbon atoms and may be represented $C_6H_{12}O_6$ (i.e. it also has 12 atoms of hydrogen, six of oxygen). In the first part of the pathway, each glucose molecule is split (via nine or 10 individual steps) into two molecules of the compound pyruvic acid, or pyruvate, which has the formula $C_3H_4O_3$: note that pyruvate is almost exactly half a glucose molecule, but with less hydrogen – that hydrogen has been taken away and can be combined with oxygen as a first step in the 'combustion' of glucose. (Pyruvic acid gets its name from the Greek for fire.) This part of the pathway is called 'glycolysis', meaning lysis, or breakdown, of glucose. This can happen in any cell in the body. The pathway was elucidated in the 1930s by the German biochemist, Otto Fritz Meyerhof, with colleagues including Gustav Embden, and is sometimes called the Embden-Meyerhof pathway. Meyerhof was later, like Krebs, a refugee from Nazi Germany, moving initially to Paris and then to the US.

If the glucose is to be completely oxidised, then the next part of this process consists of the pyruvate being consumed in the citric acid cycle, with the liberation of carbon dioxide, CO_2, and water, H_2O: two molecules of pyruvate leading to six molecules of carbon dioxide, which may be written as:

$$2\,C_3H_4O_3 + 5\,O_2 \rightarrow 6\,CO_2 + 4\,H_2O$$

So the question arises: why has evolution led us to this complicated system, when in a candle flame the glucose could be converted in one quick step into carbon dioxide and water (and heat)? The answer is key to understanding the 'point' of metabolism. During these multiple small changes, the energy that is released can be captured, not as heat, but as chemical energy that can be used for biological processes: making new cell components, doing physical work, etc. In addition, the burning of a teaspoon of glucose in a candle flame is essentially an uncontrolled process: once it starts, it's going to continue until there's no glucose left. Within a cell, on the other hand, these multiple small steps can be 'controlled': the rate at which they occur can be changed. We saw earlier that individual metabolic pathways operate at different times. Breakdown (and storage) of glucose will be especially high when plenty of sugar is available following a meal, but at other times – during fasting, for instance – there will be a need to shut down, or at least suppress, this pathway, to conserve glucose. Indeed, in the liver, the pathway can be reversed, to make new glucose when needed, from pyruvic acid and the closely related compound lactic acid. (Lactic acid gets its name from the Latin *lac* for milk, as it was first isolated from sour milk.)

Enzymes Bring about Metabolic Pathways

Each step in a metabolic pathway is a chemical reaction. These individual steps might just happen if left on their own for a long time, but might not happen very quickly, and also might go in a different direction. Metabolic steps are brought about by enzymes. An enzyme is a protein that helps the reaction to proceed in a particular way. It is what chemists would call a catalyst. We might picture this something along these lines. A molecule of glucose sticks loosely to a particular spot on a big protein molecule – let's say a paperclip attaches to a golf ball, in an indentation that is just the right shape to accept paper clips. In this position, the glucose molecule, or paper clip, is brought very close to another molecule, a drawing pin, that is stuck just adjacent (in this case, the drawing pin is a molecule of ATP, the 'energy carrier' that we will meet many times in our journey through metabolism).

The golf ball deforms just slightly and the paper clip and drawing pin 'kiss' and the sharp bit of the drawing pin (one of the three 'Ps' in ATP) gets stuck onto the paperclip (glucose molecule), which is now called glucose 6-phosphate. Because the modified paper clip is a different shape, it doesn't stick so well to the golf ball and floats off to the next step in line; likewise, the now-blunt drawing pin. A new paper clip and drawing pin can then wander along and go through the same process. The golf ball is an enzyme, and aids the conversion without being consumed itself.

When I first studied biochemistry in the early 1960s, these pathways were for the most part known in reasonable detail. There are a very large number of individual metabolic pathways. For instance, our cells have pathways for making many of the amino acids in proteins, and breaking them down. There are pathways for making the fatty substances that surround all cells, and the components of the DNA which makes up our genes. The pathways that we shall mostly be concerned with in this book are those for making, and for breaking down, fats and sugars, and to some extent amino acids (the building blocks of proteins).

To be quite frank, these pathways are a bit of a nightmare for biochemistry students. Many of them need to be learned in detail. But, as I shall explain throughout this book, the individual components of the metabolic pathways are not, for most of us, the interesting part: the interest comes from understanding how these pathways are regulated (how they change with time) and how they interact.

In 1955 Donald Nicholson, a British biochemist who taught metabolism at the University of Leeds, needed a diagram to help his students with metabolism. He created a chart showing all the then-known metabolic pathways and, importantly, where they intersected. This chart was printed by the university's architect's department. In 1960, a small biochemical firm, Koch Light, took up this project and printed and distributed the chart, which has been updated many times over the years (Figure 3.1). Most biochemical laboratories will have a copy on a wall. A colleague told me of an overseas researcher at the Hammersmith Hospital in London, studying one of these charts intently on the laboratory wall. When asked 'what are you looking for?', he answered 'I am trying to find Oxford Circus'. Indeed, a metabolic pathways chart looks very like a map of the London Underground, but far more complex. It's not surprising that students find these pathways tedious to learn.

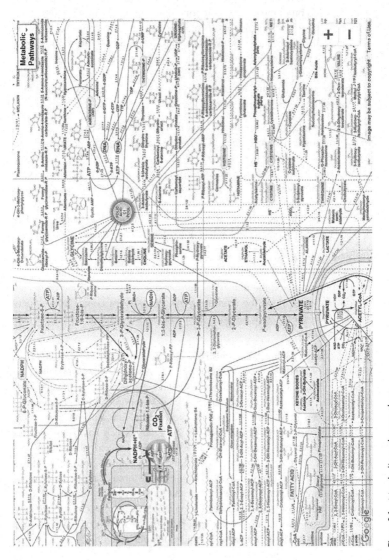

Figure 3.1   Metabolic pathways chart.

An interesting point emerges, though. Nicholson first drew his chart to teach metabolism in bacteria. And yet most of these pathways are not much different in humans. Metabolism as we now know it evolved very, very early in the development of life. A little earlier I described the action of an enzyme converting glucose to the compound glucose 6-phosphate. That enzyme is found in all cells including bacteria, fungi, plants, and animals. It has slightly different forms but is recognisably the same enzyme bringing about the same reaction.

When I was taught these pathways, they were considered to be processes operating within cells. The British biochemist Eric Newsholme pointed out that pathways, as we usually think of them, may operate not just within cells, but across different tissues. An example is this. Suppose you start to walk; your muscles need fuel. Depending on what you last ate and when, some of this will be fat that is drawn from your fat stores. So an enzyme in the fat stores somehow gets to know that your legs have started moving: fat is sent out ('mobilised') from the fat stores, through the bloodstream, to the muscles, where it can be used to derive the energy for movement. The pathway, which we might call 'fat mobilisation to provide energy for exercise', starts in one tissue and ends in another. (We might even think that, to complete the pathway, the waste products, such as carbon dioxide, need to travel through the blood and reach the lungs for breathing out.)

We continue to learn of new metabolic pathways, although now I think we can safely say that all the major metabolic pathways are known, and new discoveries tend to be 'byways', or new variations. As I have hinted, my personal interest within human metabolism has been the metabolism of fat. The technical term to cover all fats is 'lipids'. In 1971, the British biochemists Tony James and Mike Gurr published the first edition of a textbook on *Lipid Biochemistry*. This important reference book has gone through several editions. I have been a co-author since the fifth edition, which was published in 2002. More recently we have worked on the sixth edition, now called just *Lipids*, which appeared in 2016. I was pleased to find, when researching for one of my chapters on human lipid metabolism, a newly discovered pathway by which intestinal cells can get rid of cholesterol directly into the intestine. This may prove to be important in developing new drugs to treat high cholesterol levels. So there are still pathways to be discovered, although, as I mentioned, probably not major routes for the predominant compounds involved in metabolism (which we call metabolites). What is still emerging, though, and at a rapid rate, is new evidence on how metabolic pathways are regulated – i.e. how they are made to change in activity under different conditions such as feeding, fasting, and exercise.

Metabolic Pathways Go from the Twentieth to the Twenty-first Century

Studying metabolic pathways during the earlier part of the twentieth century required very careful laboratory work and many of the reagents needed had to be specially prepared, for instance by mincing up liver tissue and extracting particular enzymes. A mainstay, as the study of metabolic pathways developed, was to use a purified enzyme as a 'tool'. I will go back to the example of the enzyme that converts glucose to glucose 6-phosphate. This enzyme is commonly called hexokinase. ['Hexose' refers to the fact that it will act on most sugars that have six carbon atoms in their molecule, so-called hexoses, although glucose is the most abundant of these. 'Kinase' is a technical term meaning that the enzyme transfers a particular chemical group, known as a phosphate group, from ATP onto another molecule, thus making 'something-phosphate'. In the case of glucose, this phosphate group is added to the carbon atom conventionally known as number 6: hence the product is glucose 6-phosphate. Almost all enzymes are called 'something-ase'.]

There is another enzyme, that acts on glucose 6-phosphate, called glucose-6-phosphate dehydrogenase (as you might gather, it removes hydrogen, which is part of the process of 'combustion' since this hydrogen may then be combined with oxygen). The hydrogen is transferred to another common molecule that, like ATP, is always known by its abbreviation, in this case NADP. When NADP accepts the hydrogen, it becomes NADPH. Now it so happens that NADPH, but not NADP, absorbs ultraviolet light at a particular wavelength. So, if a biochemist wants to measure the amount of glucose in a small sample (of cell fluid, for instance, or blood, or urine) he or she may do the following: in a test-tube, add a purified form of the two enzymes (hexokinase and glucose-6-phosphate dehydrogenase), some ATP, and some NADP. She or he will place the test tube in an instrument that can shine ultraviolet light through it and measure how much comes out the other side, so showing how much of the light has been absorbed – a spectrophotometer. The biochemist then adds the sample of test fluid. The two enzymes convert glucose to glucose 6-phosphate

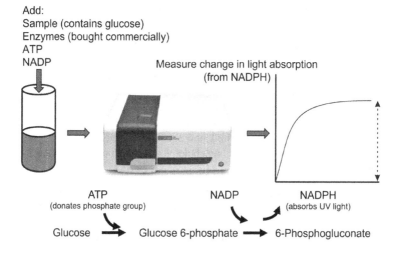

Figure 3.2 Measuring the amount of glucose in a sample using enzymes. The terms and the technique are described in the text.

and then to the slightly oxidised product, known as 6-phosphogluconate, in the process producing NADPH from NADP. The amount of UV light absorbed will increase, and then stop when the reaction is complete. By knowing how much light is absorbed for each unit weight of NADPH, the amount of glucose in the sample will be known. This is all illustrated in Figure 3.2.

Many cellular constituents can be measured in a similar way. This is known as enzymatic (or enzymic) analysis. In my laboratory we used to have on the shelf a multi-volume book called *Methods of Enzymatic Analysis*, edited by the German biochemist Hans Bergmeyer. I think our rather elderly edition had three volumes: the current edition has nine. Most of the enzymes needed for these analyses can now be bought in little bottles from specialist suppliers. This makes measurements much easier for us than they were for our predecessors. When Krebs made his discoveries of metabolic cycles, he, or his technician, would have prepared these enzymes directly for the purpose from, for instance, pieces of liver or heart (from the slaughterhouse) or from plants such as horseradish.

However, even these methods have become outdated in the twenty-first century. New techniques such as magnetic resonance spectroscopy can look at many metabolic compounds (metabolites) at one time: they produce a sort of 'fingerprint' of the metabolites present in a sample. When the sequence of the DNA making up human genes was being discovered, the term 'genomics' was invented for the study of the 'genome' (the whole complement of genes). Needless to say, biochemists now speak of the 'metabolome' for the complement of metabolites, and 'metabolomics' (sometimes metabonomics) for its study.

This ability to analyse many metabolites at once has also led to new views about the organisation of metabolic pathways within cells. It has emerged from these 'fingerprints' that there are a small number of key metabolites that are at the intersections of many pathways and may have key roles in integrating the activity of those pathways. One important metabolite like this is called acetyl-CoA, or more fully acetyl-coenzyme A. In the days before its structure was understood, it used to be called 'active acetate'. Acetate and acetic acid are essentially the same thing: dilute acetic acid is vinegar. The coenzyme A is a larger molecule that gets attached to the acetate and may facilitate it binding to enzymes and moving around the cell, like a handle. It is derived from the B vitamin pantothenic acid (vitamin B5). This structure was finally determined by yet another German biochemist who had been forced to flee with the rise of the Nazi party, Fritz Lipmann. Lipmann worked on this topic at the Massachusetts General Hospital in Boston, US, and for this work was awarded the Nobel Prize in Physiology or Medicine, which he shared with Hans Krebs (for his work on the citric acid cycle) in 1953. Acetyl-CoA will feature in our later discussions of metabolism and the 'combustion' of fuels; it is shown in Figure 3.3, although the only really important thing to note is that the acetyl, or acetate component, has two carbon atoms.

When I learned these pathways in the 1960s, I naively assumed that the metabolites were floating around inside the cell, and then by chance a paperclip and drawing pin might alight on the golf ball of hexokinase. Even then it should have been clear that this was not so, but now the evidence is stronger and stronger that there is organisation of pathways within cells, so

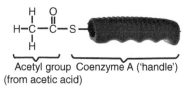

Acetyl group Coenzyme A ('handle')
(from acetic acid)

Figure 3.3 Acetyl-CoA. The acetate group, with two carbon atoms (left-hand side) is attached via an atom of sulphur (S) to a larger component called coenzyme A, which we can regard as a handle for moving it along metabolic pathways.

that a metabolite may be passed from one enzyme to another, changing step by step as it goes along. We know that some sets of enzymes are associated together with a particular component within the cell: for instance, the enzymes that bring about complete combustion are associated together on a membrane that forms part of the cellular organelle (a cell component) called the mitochondrion – of which more in Chapter 5. We have also learned that the inside of a cell is not a drop of salty water, as I might have supposed, but more like a gel, criss-crossed with protein fibres or 'microtubules' along which move little transporters, taking things to where they need to be within the cell.

I can illustrate this briefly with an example from my own laboratory. Although my own research has mainly been based upon studying whole people, we had a project later in my career looking at the metabolism of human fat cells. A PhD student in our laboratory, Jenny Collins, worked with these human fat cells to study the pathways by which they make fatty acids from sugars – a pathway that we will look at again later. This pathway is one of the 'classic pathways' of metabolism, connecting the metabolism of sugars and fats, fully worked out in the 1960s. It makes a saturated fat called palmitic acid (illustrated in Figure 2.2). Saturated fats have some detrimental effects, as you will almost certainly know from dietary advice. In the diet, they tend to raise the blood cholesterol concentration, which may increase the risk of heart disease. But cells don't do well either if they have an excess of saturated fatty acids – it may be that the regular packing of saturated fatty acids (see Figure 2.2) makes things 'too rigid'. But it turned out that the human fat cells were very good at converting these saturated fats into unsaturated, and much healthier, fats. The enzymes involved are known as desaturases. Jenny showed that palmitic acid (saturated) made from sugar was preferentially directed into desaturation – making unsaturated fat – rather than any other fate (such as oxidation). If she

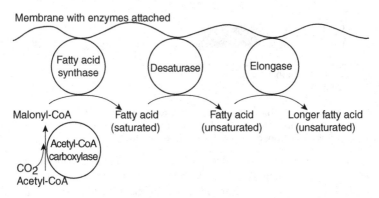

Figure 3.4 The idea of metabolic 'channelling' – metabolites are effectively passed from one enzyme to another without mixing with other components in the cell. It is illustrated here with reference to fatty acid synthesis. Based on ideas in Collins, J. M. *et al.* (2010)

added palmitic acid to the cells, it was much less likely to enter into the desaturation pathway, probably because it was not part of the same system of connected enzymes. It was clear that the product of one pathway (palmitic acid) was being effectively 'passed on' along a chain into another pathway. I have sketched how this might be in Figure 3.4. Jenny, incidentally, went on to do interesting work on fat metabolism in cancer cells.

Metabolic Pathways Underlie any Description of Human Metabolism

The study of metabolism, then, is essentially the study of the pathways that make up overall metabolism, and more especially, how they are regulated in time. This regulation of pathways requires communication between different parts of the body. So we will look at that next, followed by some more detailed explanation of the process of 'combustion', and then it will be time to see how these ideas apply to human metabolism during a typical day.

4 Communication Systems in Human Metabolism

The Need for Communication in Human Metabolism

I've been sitting at the computer for too long. It's time to go for a walk. My brain tells my leg muscles to move. This is almost instantaneous. The proteins within the muscles start using energy to contract – to slide past each other. That energy comes from ATP, the energy in which is, in turn, derived from the breakdown of nutrients. There is glycogen (carbohydrate) stored in the muscles, as we have seen, and this can sustain the contractions for a short time, but if I am going for a long, slow walk, then more fuel will be needed. As we have seen, there's lots of it in my fat stores. So a signal tells my fat stores it's time to get the enzymes in the fat cells working to break down the stored triacylglycerols, and release some fatty acids that can travel through the bloodstream to my muscles. I shall probably also need to use some glucose that my liver can produce for me from its own glycogen store. In addition, as I get going, my heart needs to beat faster to pump more blood to my muscles (to carry not just the fatty acids and glucose, but also oxygen) and to remove the waste products, in this case carbon dioxide and lactic acid, which is a breakdown product of the glucose. So there are signals racing around my body, telling particular organs and tissues to do particular things in a very coordinated way.

I've now got back and had a shower and I'm feeling pretty hungry. So I start on my lunchtime cheese sandwich. Now glucose and (more slowly) fat from the sandwich enter my bloodstream and need to be directed into breakdown or storage. Something tells my liver cells it's time to stop breaking down glycogen, and to start storing some. And something tells my fat cells the same thing for their triacylglycerol stores. My muscles will also need to rebuild their glycogen stores, depleted during my walk. Again, all this requires signals to flow, to integrate many different aspects of metabolism.

The Major Communication Systems

There are two major communication systems in our bodies that bring this about: the nervous system and the hormonal system. Each has its role in regulating metabolism, but their relative importance depends on what we are doing.

I spent the early part of my career studying metabolic changes in people who had been recently injured or were otherwise severely ill. Under those conditions, there is an overwhelming drive from the nervous system, especially the component called the sympathetic nervous system (described below), to mobilise stored fuels: part of the so-called fight or flight response. This is accompanied by secretion of the closely related hormone adrenaline (in the US called epinephrine). Something similar occurs during exercise.

Later in my career I studied people at rest or exercising gently. Then I realised that things are quite different. The hormonal systems, particularly involving the hormone insulin, take a leading role in regulating how we dispose of nutrients from the food we eat, how we store them, and then mobilise those stores as needed. But before leaving this short introduction, I need also to tell you that things in the field of hormones and metabolism are not nearly as clear as we once thought they were.

It's My Nerves ...

Nerves are sometimes described as the internet of the body. A 'nerve', as we think of it, is a structure with blood vessels and other cells, and more than one nerve cell; but the nerve cell, or neuron, is the unit that we are interested in. Nerve cells, like most cells, have a nucleus where the genes (DNA) are stored, and apparatus for making energy, but their distinguishing feature is a long projection called the axon. This may run, for instance, from the brain down the spine to reach other nerves or organs, or from the spinal cord all the way to a muscle in your big toe. The other special property of nerves is that in their membranes are proteins called 'channels' that let charged atoms, ions, through when activated in some way – principally sodium ions (Na^+) and potassium ions (K^+). These channels are made of proteins, like the glucose transporters that we met earlier. They allow an electrical voltage to travel rapidly along the axon – the 'action potential' or nerve signal.

When this signal reaches the end of the axon, it may link to another nerve, in which case usually there will be a continuation of the electrical signal along the next nerve; or the nerve may end at an organ. The nerve terminates in a structure called the synapse, and when the nerve signal reaches the synapse, a chemical messenger is released. This then acts on receptors in the next cell in line, be it another nerve or an organ. We shall look at receptors in more detail shortly (with hormones), but they are proteins that specifically bind to the chemical released from the axon, and then link to some other process in the target cell.

The human nervous system is often thought of as having four, or maybe five, components. The one we are most familiar with is the 'somatic nervous system', the nerves that run from the brain to our muscles and tell them when to contract. This is also called the 'voluntary nervous system' since we can choose when to activate it. The nerves of the somatic nervous system make contact with the muscle cells and, when a signal arrives down the nerve, lead to release of calcium ions (Ca^{2+}) within the muscle cells that start the process of contraction.

In contrast, the 'autonomic' nervous system regulates things without us having to intervene – it is the automatic control mechanism. It consists, in turn, of the sympathetic nervous system and the parasympathetic nervous system. The sympathetic nervous system acts as though 'sympathetic' to our needs: it speeds up the heart when we start to exercise, for example, and it regulates the blood pressure when we stand up after lying in bed all night. It uses a chemical called noradrenaline (norepinephrine in the US), which, as mentioned earlier, is closely related to adrenaline, to transmit its signals. The parasympathetic is the opposite of the sympathetic in many ways – it slows the heart, for instance.

There is also an 'afferent nervous system' – nerves that bring signals, such as pain, from the rest of the body back to the brain, and there is an 'enteric nervous system' that regulates our intestinal functions.

The nervous system regulates metabolism in a number of ways, some direct and some indirect. In states of stress the sympathetic nervous system can bring about mobilisation of fuels directly through nerve endings in metabolic tissues (liver and adipose tissue) – although, for completeness, I should say that there has long been debate about the latter. The difficulty is that activation of the sympathetic nervous system is always closely associated with secretion of the hormone adrenaline (epinephrine). Attempts to distinguish the two are fraught with difficulty. As an illustration, Dr Bente Stallknecht and her colleagues at the University of Copenhagen conducted studies on seven patients who were paraplegic because of spinal cord injuries. They were compared with people with an intact spinal cord. The patients had use of their arms, so they were asked to exercise by cycling with their arms. But the key point was that their sympathetic nerves didn't reach (or didn't fully reach) their lower extremities. So Bente and her colleagues looked at what happened in the fat tissue on the abdomen while the patients exercised with their arms. They were looking to see if blood flow through the tissue increased, and also the release of fatty acids: both these would normally increase during exercise to supply fuel to the working muscles. She found that, indeed, blood flow and fatty acid did increase, but not as much as in the 'intact' volunteers. But then, their levels of adrenaline in the blood were also lower. Adrenaline is released in response to nerves reaching the adrenal glands which sit above the kidneys – so the signal for releasing adrenaline was cut (at least partially) in these patients. These complicated results show just how difficult it is to answer the question of whether nerves are directly affecting metabolism.

But some things are clear. Firstly, muscle contraction, brought about by signals coming through the somatic nervous system, is a major driver of changes in metabolism: when I decide to move my muscles, whether just to get out of bed or, more purposefully, to go for a walk, energy is expended faster and metabolism must change accordingly. The sympathetic nervous system regulates much of cardiovascular function (the heart and blood vessels), and that is indirectly linked to metabolism: for instance, in order to bring oxygen and fuel to working muscles, blood flow to them must increase, which will involve both increased output from the heart and local changes opening up the blood vessels in the muscles. The function of the intestinal tract is certainly modulated by nerves, in complex ways, but with some very direct effects: for instance, signals through a big nerve of the parasympathetic nervous system called the vagus nerve, which is also involved in control of the heart, increase the secretion of acid in the stomach.

There are also indirect effects on metabolism through modulation of hormone release. There is a large body of evidence that the sympathetic and parasympathetic nervous systems change the secretion of insulin from the pancreas (of which, more shortly). Nowadays, people who get stomach ulcers linked to the production of too much stomach acid will be treated with drugs that specifically reduce acid release. (They may also get antibiotics to kill the bacteria that are involved.) But until the 1980s, when drugs first became available, one treatment for recurring ulcers was to cut the vagus nerve within the chest, so reducing stomach acid production. A number of studies of metabolism were carried out in people who had undergone this procedure. It was certainly possible to identify changes, especially in insulin production. At one time, I collected all the research papers on this topic. But, looking back, the effects were quite small and didn't affect the lives of the patients.

So now it seems appropriate to talk about hormones, since their effects on metabolism are undoubted, and profound.

Hormones Are Remarkable Signals

Hormones are signalling molecules: they are produced in one tissue, and travel through the bloodstream to influence what goes on elsewhere in the body. The word 'hormone' comes from the Greek *hormao*, meaning to urge on or excite. But the efficiency with which they may do this is quite astonishing. I will illustrate this by talking about glucose in the blood, and the hormone that undoubtedly has the major role in regulating its concentration, insulin.

To do this, I need to say more about the way we describe concentrations of substances in blood and other fluids. I have done this in Box 4.1. Do skip this if it's quite familiar.

We have already met substances that are present in blood at 'millimolar' concentrations, such as glucose, around 5 mmol/l. But earlier we met adrenaline, present in people at rest and unexcited, at about 1 nmol/l: in molar terms, 5 million times less than glucose. And yet adrenaline can regulate glucose metabolism! This is real David and Goliath stuff. How can such a tiny concentration of a signal exert so much control? I shall give you a hint shortly.

Box 4.1 Molar units.

Atoms of the different elements differ in mass. If we arbitrarily assign a value of 1 to the atoms of the lightest element, hydrogen, then a carbon atom has a mass of 12, nitrogen of 14, and oxygen of 16. These numbers are known as the 'relative atomic mass', but more commonly in the laboratory are called 'atomic weight'. We can apply the same principle to molecules. Water has molecules with two atoms of hydrogen and one of oxygen (H_2O), giving it a relative molecular mass of 18 (= $2 \times 1 + 16$). (This is often colloquially called 'molecular weight'.) Let's compare water with another liquid, alcohol, whose molecules have the composition C_2H_6O, so its relative molecular mass is 46 (= $2 \times 12 + 6 \times 1 + 16$). If you think for a moment, I hope you will see that if I compare 18 grams (g) of water with 46 g of alcohol, they will contain the same numbers of molecules. (Each molecule of alcohol is 'heavier' than each molecule of water, so we need correspondingly more grams for the same number of molecules.)

If we express the relative molecular mass in grams, then one 'molecular mass in grams' is called one gram-molecule, abbreviated 1 mole. So 18 g of water is 1 mole of water, 46 g of alcohol is 1 mole of alcohol. And 1 mole of any substance has the same number of molecules. That number is known as Avogadro's number. It is 6.0 $\times 10^{23}$. That means 6 with 23 noughts after it. It's a big number. Individual molecules are very tiny! (It is named after Amedeo Avogadro, an Italian scientist working in the late eighteenth and early nineteenth centuries.)

When I started in biochemistry, we used to measure concentrations of many things in 'mass' units. Glucose in blood, for instance, was usually measured in milligrams per 100 millilitres (mg/100 ml). A typical glucose concentration is 80–90 mg/100 ml. Cholesterol, for instance, might typically be present in blood at 190–200 mg/100 ml. Lactic acid might be present at 10 mg/100 ml. These numbers give me no feeling for the relative abundance of molecules of the substance. But if I know that the relative molecular masses of glucose, cholesterol, and lactic acid are respectively 180, 387, and 90, then I can calculate that their typical concentrations in blood would be 5, 5, and 1 millimole/litre. Immediately I have more of a feeling how they inter-relate in molecular terms. In Europe, everyone in medical sciences switched to using these 'molar' units some time quite early in my career, which means that I now think only in molar terms: I had to back-calculate to get the figures in mg/100 ml that I quoted above. But 'mass units' continue to be commonly used in the US, and are permitted by some major scientific journals. Of course, mass units can be easier in the laboratory: if I ask someone to make a solution of glucose at

5 millimole/litre they have to think a bit, whereas a solution of 180 mg/100 ml can be weighed directly. (And, whatever anyone may tell you, all we laboratory workers have at some time multiplied by the 'molecular weight' when we should have divided by it.)

We will mostly deal with things that are present in blood in 'millimolar' concentrations – as for glucose, cholesterol, and lactic acid above. Nothing in blood approaches 'molar' concentrations. The substance with the highest molar concentration in blood is sodium, present typically at about 140 millimole/litre. (To be strictly correct, that applies to sodium ions, Na^+, and the term milli-equivalents/litre should be used.) But some things are present in much lower concentrations. I shall just run over some of the smaller units here, using a solution of salt (sodium chloride, NaCl, relative molecular mass 58) to illustrate.

1 mole/litre, abbreviated 1 mol/l	58 grams/litre (abbreviated g/l)
1 millimole/litre (1 mmol/l)	58 milligrams/litre (58 mg/l) or 0.058 g/l
1 micromole/litre (1 μmol/l)	58 μg/l or 0.000058 g/l
1 nanomole/litre (1 nmol/l)	58 ng/l or 0.000000058 g/l
1 picomole/litre (1 pmol/l)	58 pg/l or 0.000000000058 g/l

Table 4.1.1   Molar concentrations. The rows go down in steps of 1 000

But before that, we will look at insulin. Insulin is a protein. It can be purified. In the early days of its use for treatment of diabetes, it was purified from the pancreas of animals killed in the slaughterhouse. It was first used in Toronto, Canada, on 23 January 1922, to treat a young boy, Leonard Thompson, who would otherwise undoubtedly have died very young from his diabetes. But the doctors who gave insulin to Leonard Thompson had some experience: their shared dog, Marjorie, had had her pancreas removed the previous November and had been living healthily with insulin treatment since then. For their work on treating diabetes with insulin, Frederick Banting and John Macleod, the head of the laboratory where the work was carried out, were awarded the

Nobel Prize in Physiology or Medicine in 1923. Banting shared his part of the prize with Charles Best, a medical student who had worked with him, and Macleod shared his with James Collip, the biochemist who had developed the procedure to purify the insulin. The results of these early trials were quite astonishing, and literally life-saving (we will consider this again in Chapter 9).

Again, the way we express measurements in the laboratory has changed. We used to measure insulin in 'units.' That is because there was, in the early days, no good chemical way to measure the amount of insulin. I am afraid that 1 unit was defined in terms of the amount that would kill half of a group of mice when injected. (And I hasten to add that such measurements were only done by the insulin manufacturers, not in laboratories such as ours.) When we measured insulin in blood, we would use as a standard, for comparison, some pure insulin that we weighed out, each batch given a 'potency' (units/mg) when produced.

But gradually the field has changed and now, as with other things in blood, we measure in molar units. A typical concentration of insulin in blood is around 50 pmol/l. (That's after fasting overnight: it will rise after breakfast.) To put that in perspective: there are 100 000 000 (100 million) times as many glucose molecules in one millilitre of blood as there are insulin molecules. I did that calculation some years ago for teaching students, but I still have to check it every time I write it, as I find it so astonishing.

You might well think that a molecule as rare as insulin can have almost nothing to do with the story of metabolism and its regulation. But how wrong you would be. It has everything to do with metabolism and regulation of metabolism. Insulin is a powerful hormone. Insulin is crucial to normal metabolism of carbohydrate, fat, and protein. Things go very wrong without it. How can such a very few molecules of a protein regulate the metabolism of so many millions more molecules of the nutrients?

Hormones and Receptors

Our view of hormones, as signals that are not themselves nutrients, is changing. As with so many areas of metabolism, as we explore more, we realise that things are not quite so simple as we once thought. When the first edition of my textbook on human metabolism appeared in 1996, it had a chapter devoted to the then-standard view of hormones. In that same year, scientists in New York described a hormone, now called leptin, produced by adipose (fat storage) tissue. Metabolism and endocrinology (the study of hormones) were beginning to merge. The latest (fourth) edition of our textbook has a large table of compounds that we have always regarded as metabolites (substances that are part of metabolism), that we now know are acting also as signals. We will consider some of those later.

But until the mid-1990s, we would have said that in general a hormone is produced by an organ or gland, and travels to another organ or tissue, where it imparts a signal but does not itself take part in further reactions. The term 'gland' means an organ that produces and liberates a substance. Some glands liberate their secretions through ducts into the outside world (e.g. salivary glands into the mouth; the pancreas liberates its digestive juices through a duct into the small intestine). Hormones don't follow such a route – they are liberated directly into the bloodstream – so you will see hormone-producing tissues referred to as 'ductless glands'. The hormone acts on its target tissue by meeting a specific receptor with which it can dock.

Hormones can take a variety of chemical forms. Insulin is a small protein. It has 51 amino acids. Incidentally, it was the first protein for which the sequence of amino acids that make it up was deciphered. This was done by Fred Sanger in Cambridge, and won him the Nobel Prize in Chemistry in 1958. (He later won a second Nobel Prize in Chemistry, in 1980, shared with Walter Gilbert, for working out how to determine the sequence of bases in DNA.) It was a difficult protein to choose. Insulin is made of two shorter chains of amino acids, joined at specific points, and also with bonds between some of the amino acids in one of the chains.

Other protein hormones include glucagon (a hormone that counters the action of insulin), and some of the sex-related hormones including follicle stimulating hormone (which encourages maturation of the sexual organs during puberty in both women and men) – strictly these are called glycoproteins, as they have multiple sugar molecules attached. Oxytocin, the 'love hormone' in the popular press, is another.

Other hormones are related to amino acids – adrenaline is derived from the amino acid tyrosine, as is thyroid hormone. And others are derived from cholesterol – the 'steroid hormones', including cortisol and sex hormones such as testosterone and oestradiol.

But all hormone receptors are proteins. The ability of proteins to adopt so many different configurations, depending on the number, order, and nature of the amino acids that make them up, makes these very specific for accepting one particular hormone, and no other (e.g. the insulin receptor).

So, to look more at insulin: this hormone is produced in specialised cells in the pancreas called the β-cells. Most of the pancreas is involved in making digestive juices (liberated through the pancreatic duct into the small intestine), but about 1–2% of the mass of the pancreas consists of clumps of cells making hormones – the islets of Langerhans, named after Paul Langerhans, a German medical student, who discovered them in 1869. (As a biochemistry student I missed a lecture on hormones and borrowed a friend's notes to catch up. It was lucky I already knew something about hormones, or I might have gone through life thinking about the eyelets of Langerhans.) The insulin-producing β-cells are found within the islets, which you can see under the microscope if you stain them appropriately (Figure 4.1).

These β-cells in the islets have a metabolic pathway that can respond to the concentration of glucose in the blood that reaches them. When the glucose concentration rises from its normal level, the β-cells release more insulin. Insulin travels round the body in the bloodstream. Because of the way the veins that leave the pancreas are arranged, insulin first reaches the liver,

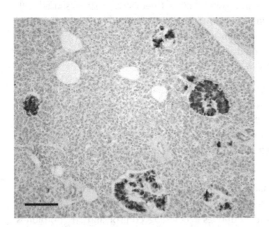

Figure 4.1   Islets of Langerhans in the pancreas.
The islets are visible in the 'sea' of exocrine tissue: insulin-containing β-cells in the islets have been identified by linking a dye to an antibody that binds to insulin. Scale bar = 100 μm (0.1 mm).

where it has effects on the liver cells, but some insulin also comes through the liver and reaches all tissues including, for instance, our muscles and our fat tissue. The cells in these tissues make a protein called the insulin receptor. It sits embedded in the membrane surrounding the cell. When insulin comes along, hormone and receptor bind together, and this initiates a change in the shape of the receptor. This shape change is translated into changes in the activity of enzymes within the cell, and hence changes in the rate at which various metabolic pathways operate.

Those last two sentences skim over the complexity of the process, and the explanation for why so very few molecules of insulin can have such a profound effect. Investigation of the mechanism by which insulin affects metabolic processes has a very long history, going back to at least the 1940s. In 1960, the first enzyme that is directly affected by insulin was discovered: it is called glycogen synthase, and is the enzyme that makes glucose units into glycogen (i.e. is responsible for storage of spare glucose). But progress was slow. There is a famous cartoon by Chuck (the pseudonym of an eminent insulin researcher, Pierre de Meyts) drawn in 1979 that characterises the state of the field at that time. A researcher in front of a blackboard says 'After years of intensive research, we finally have a clear picture of insulin action'. On the board is shown 'Insulin → Binds to receptor → Then something happens → Effects', while a little student on the floor thinks 'A long way since the black box concept'. Many people were involved in understanding this, but one key person was Philip Cohen (now Professor Sir Philip) at the University of Dundee, who discovered one of the enzymes involved. (It would take too long here to list everyone, but other researchers, especially in the US, also made contributions.) We can look at it like this. In the last chapter I described the action of an enzyme in helping a reaction to proceed – for instance, the conversion of glucose to glucose 6-phosphate. One molecule of an enzyme can bring about the reaction of a large number of molecules, maybe many tens of thousands. Imagine that the insulin receptor, having bound a molecule of insulin, now itself acts as an enzyme and modifies another enzyme (many molecules of it), which then acts on another enzyme (now many, many molecules of it), which then … until eventually the enzyme glycogen synthase itself is modified, and can then bring about the conversion of (probably) many millions of glucose molecules into glycogen. It can be seen as a 'cascade', bringing about amplification of the signal.

There Is a Large Family of G Protein-coupled Receptors

The insulin receptor, as I mentioned, sits in the membrane of the target cell. It is an unusual receptor, only loosely related to other hormone receptors. But there is a large family of hormone receptors that also sit in the cell-surface and bring about metabolic effects. These receptors all have the property that they act through a set of proteins that are called G proteins. We have met briefly the compound ATP. 'A' (adenine) is one of the bases in DNA; another is guanine, G, and there is also a compound GTP, guanosine triphosphate. G proteins are so-called because they involve GTP in their action. These receptors, known as the G protein-coupled receptors, are widespread and incredibly important for many aspects not just of metabolism, but also of cardiovascular function, and in other areas of human health. Many of them are now the targets for drugs: it has been estimated that around 30% of all drugs on the market are aimed at these receptors. An important class of G protein-coupled receptors are those that respond to adrenaline and nor-adrenaline (these act through the same receptors), called adrenergic receptors or adrenoceptors. Again, these form a large family, but are broadly categor-ised into α-adrenergic receptors and β-adrenergic receptors. β-adrenergic receptors tend to bring about fuel mobilisation and effects needed for 'fight or flight' situations, for instance increased heart output, whereas α-adrenergic receptors tend to do the opposite.

Adrenaline is a hormone released from the adrenal glands. There are two of these glands; one sits above each of the kidneys. Adrenaline is released in response to any sort of stress, and usually its release parallels increased activity of the sympathetic nervous system (mediated through noradrenaline). How do the adrenal glands know when to secrete adrenaline? They are acted upon by nerves that come down the spinal cord, so bringing signals directly from the brain. Adrenaline and noradrenaline are made by the same pathway from the amino acid tyrosine, but there is one further metabolic step in making adrenaline compared with noradrenaline – it has an extra group, a 'methyl group' ($-CH_3$) added. The enzyme that brings that about is found only in the adrenal gland, not in sympathetic nerves.

Insulin leads to an increase in glycogen formation from glucose – it is a 'storage' hormone. Adrenaline, acting through β-adrenergic receptors in the liver, can stimulate an enzyme that breaks glycogen down to liberate glucose.

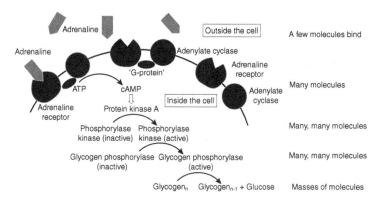

Figure 4.2 Activation of glycogen breakdown by adrenaline.

So it has the opposite effect – it is a 'fuel mobilising hormone'. The signal chain that links adrenaline binding to its receptor to the activation of glycogen breakdown was the first complete such chain to be elucidated. It illustrates a number of important mechanisms, so we will look at it here (see Figure 4.2). Key to this is a process within cells for modifying a protein by adding to one of its amino acids a phosphate group, taken from an ATP molecule. As in the case of hexokinase, the enzyme that transfers a phosphate group from ATP to glucose, this transfer is also brought about by an enzyme called a kinase. The general term for such an enzyme is a protein kinase. Adding a phosphate group changes the electrical charge on that amino acid, and may change the conformation of the protein chain, in turn – if the protein is an enzyme – altering its enzymatic activity. This mechanism for changing the activity of an enzyme is ubiquitous in all life forms. There are some protein kinase enzymes that can act on a wide range of target proteins, others that are quite specific to one target protein.

The enzyme that breaks down glycogen to liberate glucose is called glycogen phosphorylase (because it uses phosphate groups, yet again, to split off the glucose units). It is activated by phosphorylation on some key amino acids in its chain, making 'active' glycogen phosphorylase (also called glycogen phosphorylase *a*). The enzyme that brings this about is called phosphorylase kinase (i.e. it is a kinase, transferring phosphate from ATP to the enzyme glycogen phosphorylase). But in turn, believe it or not, phosphorylase kinase is itself activated by accepting a phosphate group from ATP through the action of a kinase: in this case, a general protein kinase called protein kinase A. Protein kinase A is activated by a small molecule made from ATP called cyclic AMP (usually abbreviated cAMP) in which the three phosphate groups from which ATP gets its name (adenosine triphosphate) interact, two of them are lost, and the remaining one forms a link back to the adenosine base (so making a cyclic molecule). This cAMP, in turn, is made by the enzyme adenylate cyclase, which is embedded in the cell membrane and linked to the β-adrenergic receptors through a G-protein. It sounds complicated, although it is slightly less so than the signal chain by which insulin brings about its effects.

Some Receptors Affect the Synthesis of Proteins from Genes

There is another large group of hormone receptors that are not found on the surface of the cells, but instead inside the cell, sometimes associated with the nucleus (where the DNA is stored). These act in a different way, not through a cascade of enzymes. Examples are the receptor for cortisol (called the glucocorticoid receptor) and the receptor for thyroid hormone. Because the receptors are inside the cells, the respective hormone must first itself get through the cell membrane, usually with the aid of a protein that forms a specific channel for it. Once the hormone has met and bonded with its receptor, they migrate to the nucleus of the cell, where they interact directly with the DNA, binding to specific regions, to cause particular genes to be expressed – that is, read off as RNA which can be translated into protein. This is a completely different mechanism from those we have met before, in which an enzyme was modified to change its activity. That latter process can be extremely rapid (within seconds in some cases). But binding to the DNA, causing messenger RNA to be produced, which then leaves the nucleus and serves as the code for making new proteins, is a much slower process – typically taking a matter of hours, if not days. With regard to metabolism, this is typically a mechanism for bringing about long-term changes. An example might be that if I were to read an article in the newspaper that suggested I ought to eat a Mediterranean diet, or anything else, and I were to change my eating habits, then that would bring about a gradual change – or adaptation – of the enzymes I have available to deal with it, over a period perhaps of several days. The contrast is with my setting out for a brisk walk, and within less than a minute I am using my glycogen stores, my heart is beating faster and my muscles are receiving more blood.

Metabolism and Hormones Begin to Get Confused

I mentioned earlier the hormone leptin, discovered the same year, 1996, that the first edition of my textbook on metabolism appeared. Now, needless to say, the chapter on hormones has been much revised. Leptin is produced, not by a classic 'ductless gland', but by adipose tissue, the tissue in which we store our fat reserves. It is indeed the adipocytes themselves, the fat-storing cells, that make and secrete leptin. Leptin acts on the brain – so this is a reversal of the common route of signals coming from the brain to influence 'metabolic tissues.' The bigger the fat cells get – the more fat they are storing – the more leptin they produce. And then leptin signals this fact to the brain, which tries to respond by reducing appetite.

Other tissues that we thought were concerned with metabolism are now known to produce hormones. The kidneys produce hormones that regulate blood pressure; the intestines produce hormones that regulate digestion and perhaps again appetite; the heart produces a hormone that regulates salt loss via the kidneys; there is even evidence (still a little controversial) that muscles release hormones that influence inflammation and perhaps delivery of fatty acids from fat tissue during exercise.

But now there is another complication. It turns out that a number of substances that we think of as being involved in metabolism can also act as signals via the G protein-coupled receptors in cell membranes.

Dr Derek Williamson was the successor to Hans Krebs as head of the Metabolic Research Laboratory in Oxford. Derek Williamson was an enormously productive biochemist who studied many aspects of metabolism, but had a particular interest in fat metabolism, mainly studying this in cells and in laboratory animals. When fatty acids are broken down in the liver, they may not be completely combined with oxygen: some may emerge as intermediate compounds called ketone bodies. We shall examine ketone bodies much more when we talk about metabolism in starvation. The metabolic pathway for making ketone bodies was elucidated in the 1940s, so they and their metabolism were well known when Derek had his interest in them, from the 1960s onwards. Derek always had a feeling that the ketone bodies were something more than a partial breakdown product of fat, able to be used for energy by other tissues than the liver. He thought they carried a signal. Indeed, in 1980 he published an article in the influential journal *Physiological Reviews* with a colleague, Alison Robinson, entitled 'Physiological roles of ketone bodies as substrates and signals in mammalian tissues'. But the G protein-coupled receptors were hardly known then, and Derek could not have taken this further. Very sadly for all who knew him, and for the metabolism community at large, Derek died young, just after retirement. The second edition of my textbook on metabolism, published in 2003, was dedicated to Derek and to Denis McGarry, two metabolic scientists who both worked on fatty acids and ketone bodies, knew each other well, and both of whom died young.

But since then, Derek's ideas have been fully vindicated. To explain how, we need to know about a rather old treatment for high lipid levels (cholesterol and triacylglycerol) in the blood, using the compound niacin, or vitamin B3, in high doses. This treatment is known to reduce blood lipid levels at least in part by reducing fatty acid release from fat cells (adipocytes). The mechanism, though, was not understood until modern techniques were applied in the twenty-first century. In 2003, two groups independently identified a receptor for niacin. This receptor is a G protein-coupled receptor, now called GPR109A. Niacin in the concentrations needed to lower lipid levels is not a normal constituent of the blood, so this suggested that some other substance was the real partner for GPR109A. Further investigation showed that GPR109A is activated by one of the ketone bodies, called 3-hydroxybutyrate, at concentrations that might realistically be found in the blood. Since GPR109A is present in fat cells (adipocytes), this makes an elegant metabolic control mechanism: fat cells release fatty acids, which are used by the liver; the liver in turn releases ketone bodies; these can then signal through GPR109A to the fat cells to reduce fatty acid release. So the system is self-limiting.

Since that time, a large number of other metabolic substances, including fatty acids, have been shown to affect metabolism by binding to specific G protein-coupled receptors. So, as I said, the old distinctions between metabolism and endocrinology are fast being blurred.

With our new understanding of these control systems regulating metabolism, and after a look at the cellular mechanisms for deriving energy from nutrients, we can begin to look at how metabolism changes during our normal daily lives.

5 ATP: The Common Currency of Metabolic Energy

The Idea of an 'Energy Currency'

I know I am not alone in my fascination with steam engines. The steam engine is an external combustion engine. The fuel burns in the firebox. It produces heat. The heat is then used to generate steam in the boiler. The steam, under pressure, is then piped to the cylinders where it acts to move the pistons and hence to do work like moving a ship through water, or an engine along the rails, or, in the case of a stationary pumping engine, lifting water out of a deep mine. So the steam is a way of transferring the energy liberated when the fuels are burned, to the place where energy is needed to do work.

Similarly, in the cell, nutrients are oxidised in discrete structures called mitochondria (singular, mitochondrion). Instead of steam, something else is produced: ATP. ATP is adenosine triphosphate (sometimes adenosine trisphosphate in biochemical literature). So the mitochondrion, often called the powerhouse of the cell, is like firebox and boiler. Now, just as steam may be led to the working parts of the machinery through pipes, ATP can move around the cell to where it is needed. And, if we take muscles as analogous to engines, ATP can drive the contraction of a muscle just as steam can move a piston and do work.

This will be the last of our chapters mainly on cellular metabolism. We will explore the concept of the 'final common pathway' for oxidation of nutrients, and the wonderful simplicity of the citric acid, or Krebs, cycle which underlies the provision of energy for organisms from daisies, through butterflies, to you and me. By understanding how all energy-providing nutrients feed into the same pathway, we shall be better able to understand how they relate to each other – for instance, whether it makes any difference whether we take in our energy mainly as alcohol, carbohydrate, fat, or protein.

What Is ATP?

The famous double helix that is the basis of DNA structure is made of two chains composed of alternating sugar molecules and phosphate groups. Attached to the sugar molecules are the four bases, meaning substances that would, on their own, be somewhat alkaline. These are adenine, guanine, cytosine and thymine, abbreviated A, G, C, and T. They face the centre of the helix, each linking loosely to a complementary base on the other strand (A with T, C with G), and their sequence encodes the information for the synthesis of proteins, in genes in the DNA. (Each consecutive set of three bases codes for one particular amino acid, to be added to a protein.) The unit of a sugar linked to one of the bases is called a nucleoside. When phosphate groups attach to the sugar, it is called a nucleotide.

In DNA, the sugar involved is a five-carbon sugar, ribose, but missing one of the oxygen atoms that would normally be present. So it is called deoxyribose. DNA is deoxyribonucleic acid (it contains deoxyribose, it's found in the nucleus, and it is acidic in solution, because of the phosphate groups). In the related molecule RNA, which carries the code from the DNA gene to the machinery that reads it off and makes proteins, the sugar is ribose. RNA is ribonucleic acid. (There are several types of RNA, but the one I mentioned is called messenger RNA, or mRNA.)

The ATP involved in energy provision is the same as the nucleotide building block of RNA – it has adenine (A) attached to the sugar ribose, and attached to the ribose are three 'phosphate groups'. Its molecular structure is shown in Figure 5.1, to help you envisage what we are talking about. ATP is made from adenosine monophosphate, AMP (one phosphate group), via the intermediate adenosine diphosphate, ADP (two phosphate groups). This link between genes and energy transfer perhaps shows something about the evolution of metabolism – it would be wasteful to develop a completely different compound when one exists already in the genetic material.

We have met 'phosphate groups' before. They are commonly transferred onto proteins to change their structure – and, indeed, to change their activity in the case of enzymes (e.g. glycogen phosphorylase, the enzyme that removes

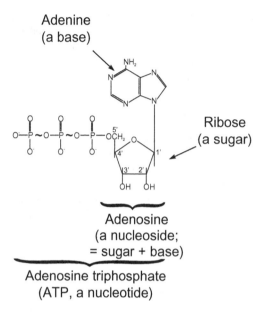

Figure 5.1   The structure of ATP.
The three phosphate groups are on the left. The 'high-energy' bonds between phosphate groups are shown as 'squiggles' (~), to be discussed shortly.

glucose units from glycogen). They are also transferred onto metabolic compounds such as glucose, in that case making glucose 6-phosphate which then enters metabolic pathways in the cell. These phosphate groups are derived from phosphoric acid, H_3PO_4. The phosphate group, when attached to another compound such as glucose, can be written as $-H_2PO_3$, or to be strictly accurate, since this is an acidic group and the hydrogen atoms will be dissociated as hydrogen ions (H^+), it is written as $-PO_3^{2-}$ (plus 2 H^+). However, the phosphate group is conveniently shown in molecular structures as $-Ⓟ$.

There is something special about the second and third phosphate groups in ATP. Forming the bond that joins them to the rest of the molecule needs more energy than the first phosphate group's bond, and conversely, more energy is released when it is broken. These bonds are often called 'high-energy bonds' although purists in thermodynamics criticise that term – but it's a useful way of thinking. The German-American biochemist Fritz Lipmann, mentioned in Chapter 3 as the discoverer of coenzyme A, introduced a nomenclature for this, generally called the 'squiggle bond', thus: Adenosine-P~P~P, where the squiggles show the bonds that release more energy when broken.

Metabolism and Combustion

In Chapter 1, we saw Antoine Lavoisier's conclusion that '*La respiration est donc une combustion*'. As we have seen, within cells, glucose, fats, and amino acids are not actually burned, but are broken down by a series of small steps, that lead ultimately to the same end-products as burning: carbon dioxide and water. The reason for this – apart from the obvious that we don't want our cells to catch fire – is that the laws of thermodynamics mean that more of the energy can be 'captured' in a useful form other than heat. Indeed, as adult humans, we do not use fuels primarily to generate heat – we get plenty of heat as a by-product of metabolism. We use fuels to do other things – physical work is an obvious example, but also making new compounds (e.g. new proteins), keeping the brain thinking, and generally keeping all our cells working. And, to a very large extent, this means that within a cell, the energy from breaking fuels down is captured by making ATP, which can then be used for many cellular processes – all those just listed, and many others.

Two Ways of Making ATP

When we talk about 'making ATP' or 'synthesising ATP' in the cell, we are not talking about making anything from scratch. There is, indeed, a metabolic pathway for making 'A', adenine, although we also obtain it from food. But usually when we think of a cell making ATP to use for some purpose that requires energy, we are simply talking about adding together the diphosphate form, ADP, and a phosphate group. The enzyme that makes most of the ATP, and was the subject of research that led to several Nobel Prizes (as we shall see later in this chapter), is called ATP synthase. And yet it does nothing more than add together ADP and 'P'. And where have these come from? From ATP, when it has been used to provide energy. The components are simply being recycled (Figure 5.2).

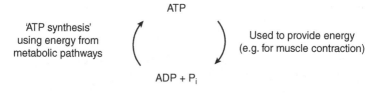

Figure 5.2   Synthesis of ATP is more properly seen as recycling.
P_i ('inorganic phosphate') is the nomenclature for an isolated phosphate group.

Some ATP can be made directly in reactions that we have already met. In glycolysis, the initial pathway for glucose breakdown in which glucose is converted to pyruvic acid, there are steps in the chain in which the enzyme involved uses ADP and makes ATP directly. This way of making ATP is called 'substrate level phosphorylation' (phosphorylation here means adding a phosphate group to ADP, as shown in Figure 5.2). ATP is also *used* in glycolysis. (We have seen that the first step is converting glucose to glucose 6-phosphate, and this uses one molecule of ATP, releasing ADP. A further molecule of ATP is used at a subsequent step.) Overall, in converting one molecule of glucose to pyruvic acid, two molecules of ATP are used, and four are made: net gain, 2 ATP. If the pyruvic acid is converted then to lactic acid, we have the overall reaction $C_6H_{12}O_6$ (glucose) $\rightarrow$ 2 $C_3H_6O_3$ (lactic acid) and a net gain of 2 ATP. This pathway does not need oxygen, and is the route for making ATP in tissues that do not use much oxygen, or that cannot use oxygen (e.g. red blood cells). It is also the pathway used by muscles at the beginning of exercise, before blood flow and heart pumping have increased to bring more oxygen and remove carbon dioxide.

However, much, much more ATP can be produced when oxygen comes into play. Here is the difference, though, from combustion. In combustion, the glucose, or fat, interacts with oxygen directly. For glucose, the chemical reaction would be written as:

$$C_6H_{12}O_6 + 6O_2 \rightarrow 6CO_2 + 6H_2O \quad (+\text{heat liberated})$$

In metabolism, oxygen is used in a separate compartment of the cell: the mitochondrion. And much of the energy that would be liberated as heat in burning is, instead, captured as chemical energy in the molecule of ATP.

Mitochondria

Mitochondria are structures, organelles, within cells. Most human cells have mitochondria – there are only a few exceptions, red blood cells being an important one. So do plant cells, incidentally, as well as insect cells, but not bacteria. Mitochondria must have developed early in evolutionary terms. There may be few or many mitochondria, depending on the nature of the cell. Muscle cells, including heart muscle, have many that help them achieve high rates of energy generation. The specialised tissue, brown adipose tissue, which makes heat in small animals, has plenty of mitochondria in order to oxidise fuels to make heat. 'Ordinary' (or 'white') adipose tissue, the fat storage tissue, on the other hand, has cells with relatively few mitochondria, since its main function of storing and mobilising fat does not need much energy.

Mitochondria are usually described as lozenge-shaped, although they can take many forms. When I studied biochemistry in the 1960s, an idea was emerging that mitochondria represented simpler organisms, bacteria or something similar, that had at some point merged with more complex cells. There were a number of reasons for believing this. Mitochondria have their own DNA, encoding some of the proteins that they need – although other mitochondrial proteins are encoded by genes in the cell's nucleus. A strong argument for their separate origin was that the apparatus for making proteins from the message in RNA was more similar to the bacterial apparatus than to that of more complex organisms. There were also suggestions that mitochondria could be seen dividing to make new mitochondria, just as bacteria might do – difficult to prove, though, in those days, as the idea was mostly based on snapshot photographs using the electron microscope, not real-time observation of the process of division. In the intervening years, the idea of a separate origin for mitochondria has been completely accepted. It is known as endosymbiosis. At some time in the distant past, a bacterium or something similar took up residence in another cell, and they both benefitted from the arrangement. The resulting cells, that I have been calling 'more complex', are what we call eukaryotic cells – the basis of all plants, fungi, and animals – major features distinguishing them from prokaryotic cells (bacteria and archaea) being the presence of mitochondria, and that the DNA is stored in chromosomes in a nucleus. Figure 5.3 shows the structure of a mitochondrion.

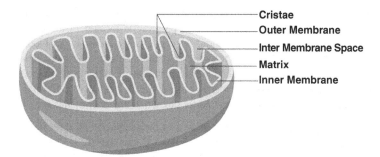

Figure 5.3   A mitochondrion.

Each mitochondrion is surrounded by a double membrane. The inner membrane is folded inwards making projections called cristae, which increase the surface area. The space between the membranes is important for their function, but most of the action goes on within the inner space (called the mitochondrial matrix) and on the inner surface of the inner membrane.

Cellular Location of Metabolic Pathways

Most of the key pathways for breaking nutrients down are situated within the mitochondrion. In contrast, pathways for making nutrients (glucose, fatty acids, even cholesterol) happen outside the mitochondrion, in the cell cytoplasm. This is a form of 'compartmentation' – separation of different functions in the same cell.

This separation of pathways may have evolved to provide more control over the individual pathways. Take fat oxidation, for example: fatty acids are broken down into units of two carbon atoms (in fact to the now-familiar acetyl-CoA; see Figure 3.3) in the mitochondria. But the pathway for making fatty acids from 2-carbon units (again, acetyl-CoA) is situated in the cytoplasm. If they were sitting side by side, one could imagine that a cycle might occur with breakdown to acetyl-CoA and then resynthesis – using energy but not achieving anything.

But some pathways of breakdown are split between the cytoplasm and the mitochondrion. We have looked at the pathway of glycolysis, whereby glucose is split in half, producing two molecules each with three carbon atoms in the form of pyruvic acid. This pathway is located in the cell's cytoplasm, not in the mitochondrion. (Hence it can operate in red blood cells, which lack mitochondria.) Pyruvic acid can then enter the mitochondria – there is a transporter protein in the membrane, with 'pyruvate-shaped holes'. The outer mitochondrial membrane is generally more permeable than the inner, so these transporters are mostly situated in the inner membrane.

Oxidation to liberate energy is the process of breaking apart all the carbon atoms so they can be combined with oxygen, O_2, to make carbon dioxide, CO_2, which can then be expelled via the lungs. It will be useful here to list the numbers of carbon atoms in the molecules of the substances we are dealing with. Glucose, as we have seen, has six carbon atoms in each molecule. Pyruvic acid, being almost half a glucose molecule, has three.

Once pyruvate is inside the mitochondrion, it has two possible fates. The choice will depend upon the metabolic and nutritional state (so hormones, especially insulin, will control it). If the body is short of glucose (e.g. when fasting), then pyruvate can be 'salvaged' to convert back to glucose (so six carbons – glucose – went to 2 × three carbons; now they can recombine to make new glucose). That's the pathway called gluconeogenesis (making new glucose), and occurs in the cytoplasm of liver cells. It makes glucose which can be released into the bloodstream. But the other fate of pyruvate, when there is plenty of carbohydrate available, is to enter the pathway of complete oxidation. And the first step here is the action of an enzyme called pyruvate dehydrogenase. Its name suggests that it removes hydrogen atoms from pyruvic acid. And removal of hydrogen atoms is equivalent to oxidation, because these hydrogen atoms can move to somewhere where oxygen is available and react together to make water ({H} atoms + O_2 → H_2O).

Pyruvate dehydrogenase is a complex enzyme, consisting of three separate enzymes acting together (it is often called PDC, pyruvate dehydrogenase complex). Another of the enzymes in the complex removes one carbon atom from the pyruvic acid, so now we have a molecule with two carbon atoms: it is effectively acetic acid (like vinegar), but it becomes linked to the larger molecule called coenzyme A, making acetyl-CoA. (The coenzyme A component we can envisage like a handle as shown in Figure 3.3 – it's the acetyl part with two carbon atoms that we are following here.) I have said before that acetyl-CoA is a key intermediate in many metabolic pathways – shortly we shall see the relevance of this.

Before looking at oxidation directly, we will look at another pathway that is split between cytoplasm and mitochondrion: that of alcohol breakdown.

Alcohol Metabolism

Alcohol, as we drink it, is the compound chemists call ethanol. The term alcohol refers, chemically, to a compound whose molecules have a free hydroxyl (–OH) group. Molecules of ethanol have two carbon atoms, with the hydroxyl group attached to one: its formula is C_2H_6O. Acetic acid, which can become acetyl-CoA, has the formula $C_2H_4O_2$. So compared with ethanol, acetic acid has less hydrogen, and more oxygen – it is a (partially) oxidised form of ethanol. In liver cells, there are two oxidation steps converting ethanol to acetic acid, which can then be converted to acetyl-CoA. The first of the oxidation steps, brought about by alcohol dehydrogenase, occurs in the cytoplasm, making acetaldehyde (C_2H_4O). Acetaldehyde in our tissues is thought to be the main reason for the feeling of a 'hangover' after drinking alcohol. Then the acetaldehyde moves into the mitochondria for the next oxidation step, conversion to acetic acid and then acetyl-CoA, brought about by acetaldehyde dehydrogenase. The hydrogen atoms removed in this process can be transferred within the mitochondrion for combination with oxygen.

So breakdown of alcohol, like glucose – and, as we shall see, fat and many of the amino acids – leads to acetyl-CoA, which can feed into the citric acid cycle along with other metabolic fuels (although alcohol breakdown is almost entirely confined to liver cells).

Fatty Acid Breakdown

In contrast to glucose metabolism, the first stage of which happens outside the mitochondrion (in the cytoplasm), fatty acid breakdown occurs entirely within the mitochondrion. When fatty acids enter a cell, the first step in their metabolism, whatever their ultimate fate, is to link them to the 'handle' of coenzyme A. This step is often called 'activation', since it prepares the fatty acid for further metabolism. This happens as they enter the cell and there is evidence in some cells that this process, brought about by enzymes called acyl-CoA synthases, is intimately linked to the transport of fatty acids into the cells. (The term 'acyl' in acyl-CoA refers to the acid, as in fatty acid; sometimes it is spelled out as fatty acyl-CoA.)

But fatty acyl-CoA molecules cannot cross the mitochondrial membrane. There is a complex process whereby the coenzyme A is replaced with the small, polar molecule carnitine, and the acyl-carnitine molecule is transported into the mitochondrion, where the carnitine is in turn replaced by coenzyme A. I mention this complication because this step, entry of the fatty acid molecule into the mitochondrion, is a key step for regulation. We will look at this in detail in Chapter 8.

When I described fatty acids in Chapter 2, I gave examples such as palmitic acid, with 16 carbons, and oleic acid, with 18. Almost all fatty acids in mammals have even numbers of carbon atoms in their molecules. The reason is simple. The pathway for making fatty acids, in plants and animals, involves sequential additions of 2-carbon units in the form of acetyl-CoA (which might have come from glucose, or even alcohol). Therefore the resultant fatty acids have even numbers of carbon atoms. Bacteria have different patterns of fatty acid metabolism. Most of us will have a few odd-numbered fatty acids (e.g. with 15 or 17 carbon atoms) in our tissues, because bacteria within cows' intestines partially break the fatty acids down, making odd-numbered fatty acids, which can be incorporated into dairy products and hence into our own tissues.

The pathway for breaking down fatty acids also occurs through stepwise removal of 2-carbon units, each time making one molecule of acetyl-CoA. It is often shown as a spiral – the fatty acyl-CoA molecule shuttles between different enzymes, which cut the chain of carbon atoms two behind the 'head' (acid) group. That carbon atom is known as the β-carbon, so this pathway is called β-oxidation. After removal of two carbon atoms from the chain, the now-shortened fatty acid repeats the sequence, until it has all been cut up into 2-carbon units in the form of acetyl-CoA.

Note the difference: one molecule of glucose makes two molecules of acetyl-CoA, whereas one molecule of, say, oleic acid (18 carbons) makes nine molecules of acetyl-CoA – fatty acids are, as we have seen, a potent source of energy.

Many Amino Acids also Lead to Acetyl-CoA

I have noted already that there is great variety amongst the 20 amino acids commonly found in proteins, but some of them also follow pathways of breakdown that lead to acetyl-CoA. So acetyl-CoA is a common intermediate in pathways of breakdown of nutrients.

This is an opportunity to look at another aspect of the breakdown of amino acids. Each amino acid, by definition, includes an amino group $(-NH_2)$ which contains a nitrogen atom. So, unlike sugars and fatty acids, amino acids cannot be completely oxidised to CO_2 and water. A possible product of breakdown would be ammonia, NH_3, but this is very toxic. Aquatic animals excrete the nitrogen resulting from amino acid breakdown mainly as ammonia, since there is plenty of water around to dilute it. Land-dwelling animals, including mammals, mostly excrete this nitrogen in a different form, urea (CN_2H_4O). Compared with ammonia, this is much less toxic (so needs to be diluted with much less water), and each molecule carries away two atoms of nitrogen. (Some animals, including birds, excrete nitrogen as uric acid.) Urea is formed in another metabolic cycle, also discovered by Hans Krebs, called the urea cycle: essentially, amino acids transfer their nitrogen atoms from one to another and they can then enter the urea cycle in the liver. Urea travels through the bloodstream to the kidneys, where it is excreted in urine.

The Fate of Acetyl-CoA

Acetyl-CoA is indeed at the central cross-roads of many pathways of metabolism. Some are shown in Figure 5.4.

But here we are going to look at one particular fate of acetyl-CoA: its entry into the citric acid cycle – the bottom arrow in Figure 5.4. This, as we shall see, leads to its complete breakdown to carbon dioxide. So we see that glucose, fatty acids, some amino acids, and alcohol converge at acetyl-CoA on their way to complete breakdown.

Oxidation and the Citric Acid (Krebs) Cycle

The meaning of 'oxidation' is combination with oxygen. In the case of molecules such as those we meet in metabolism, containing carbon, oxygen, and hydrogen atoms, this will mean breaking them apart to release carbon

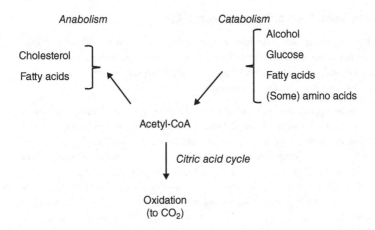

Figure 5.4   Acetyl-CoA at the centre of the metabolic network.
The right-hand side shows the flow of carbon atoms from nutrients into oxidation (via the citric acid/Krebs cycle). The left shows how acetyl-CoA can also be used to make new substances – e.g. glucose might make acetyl-CoA, which is then used to make fatty acids or cholesterol. Note the parallels with the diagram of catabolism and anabolism in Figure 1.3.

dioxide, CO_2, and water, H_2O. (Amino acids are a little different because they all, by definition, also contain nitrogen atoms (N). As we have seen, this nitrogen is converted in the liver to the relatively harmless product urea, and then excreted in the urine.)

In our cells, oxidation may mean removal of hydrogen atoms, and then these hydrogen atoms can later, in a separate place, combine with oxygen. (I will show these hydrogen atoms 'in transit' as {H}.) These hydrogen atoms are carried in the cell by one of the universal 'hydrogen carriers' – they have a role rather like ATP as the universal energy carrier. The most common is called NAD (nicotinamide-adenine dinucleotide). In its oxidised form, it is written NAD; when it accepts two hydrogen atoms it becomes the reduced form, written $NADH_2$. [In modern biochemistry texts a slightly different, but less obvious, notation is used: NAD^+ and NADH (+ H^+).] These two hydrogen atoms can then, at a later stage, be transferred to oxygen:

$$4\{H\} + O_2 \rightarrow 2H_2O$$

and so, effectively, the compound that donated the {H} to the NAD is now itself oxidised.

So now we are heading rapidly towards the central pathway of oxidative metabolism – the citric acid, or Krebs, cycle, named after its discoverer. This is the mechanism by which acetyl-CoA (with its two carbon atoms) is oxidised. Incidentally, when Krebs was doing most of his work, the nature of acetyl-CoA was not recognised. The substance was referred to as 'active acetate'. Krebs, in many of his papers from this time (late 1930s/early 1940s), described the pathway for the 'oxidation of pyruvate', since that was often his starting point.

The citric acid cycle works as follows. The acetyl component of acetyl-CoA (with two carbon atoms) joins with a 4-carbon molecule called oxaloacetate, making a compound with six carbon atoms in its molecules. This compound is citric acid. It is the same citric acid that gives citrus fruits their tartness. It has three 'carboxylic acid' groups (-COOH), making it an acid, and this gives the process its other widely used name: the tricarboxylic acid cycle. Then a series of reactions follows (each brought about by a specific enzyme, within the mitochondrion) during which carbon atoms are sequentially removed in the form of carbon dioxide, CO_2, and 'reducing equivalents' (effectively hydrogen atoms) are transferred elsewhere to meet their fate of combination with oxygen. After two carbon atoms have been lost, we have a compound with four carbon atoms in its molecules, which then becomes oxaloacetate again – ready to combine with another molecule of acetyl-CoA, and so the cycle begins anew. This is illustrated in Figure 5.5.

The citric acid cycle (that's the term that Krebs himself used) is universal amongst living organisms. It is beautiful in its simplicity. And it is the 'final common pathway' for oxidation of all the nutrients that give us energy. Almost all our cells have it, although there are a few, such as red blood cells, that do not, as they have no mitochondria.

How should we envisage this cycle? We know that the enzymes and their products do not float around in the mitochondrial matrix. We know that, in part, because of experiments with radioactive isotope labelling, which show that citric acid must be transferred from one enzyme to another without floating free – if it floated free, its symmetry would determine that the next carbon dioxide to be lost could come from either end, whereas in fact it always comes from one particular end. (See Figure 3.4 for an illustration of

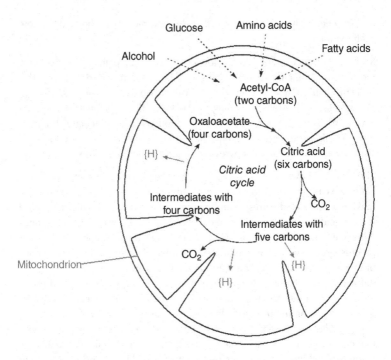

Figure 5.5 The citric acid (or Krebs) cycle in outline. Nutrients are broken down to acetyl-CoA (with two carbon atoms) within the mitochondria. Acetyl-CoA combines with oxaloacetate, a compound with four carbon atoms, to make citric acid. Sequential oxidation (removing 'reducing equivalents', or hydrogen atoms, shown here as {H}) and removal of two carbon atoms as CO_2 brings the cycle back to oxaloacetate, ready to combine with another molecule of acetyl-CoA.

how this might be.) Some enzymes of the cycle can be shown experimentally to be physically linked to each other, and in reality they are probably clustered together in some functional way, bound at least loosely to the inner membrane of the mitochondrion.

Oxidative Phosphorylation

Some ATP is made directly in the citric acid cycle by substrate-level phosphorylation – I have not shown that, for simplicity. Most is made when the hydrogen atoms, carried by $NADH_2$ and other carriers, are combined with oxygen. This happens in a series of linked enzymes embedded in the inner mitochondrial membrane, called the electron transport chain. ('Electrons' here are reducing equivalents, effectively the same as hydrogen atoms, {H}.) During this transfer of reducing equivalents, they are combined with oxygen, so releasing energy. And the cell traps most of this energy by making ATP via the enzyme ATP synthase (which, as we saw, simply adds 'P' to ADP).

When I studied biochemistry, we were taught that the electron transport chain led to the build-up of some high-energy-containing intermediate compound, whose energy could then be used to make ATP. The nature of this intermediate was unclear. But we were also told in passing about a rogue scientist, Peter Mitchell, who had a different theory about how ATP is made. Peter Mitchell was a biochemist who, in 1961, promoted a theory known as the chemiosmotic theory for how cells make ATP. These views went against mainstream thinking, and Mitchell, who had independent means, bought and renovated a Georgian manor house, Glynn House, on Bodmin Moor in Cornwall, and created his own laboratories. There, with a research group of only three or four people, he toiled away, collecting evidence to support his contention. For many years he remained isolated from the scientific mainstream. But then, gradually, other scientists began to appreciate that Mitchell might have got a point; and, following gradual and sometimes unwilling acceptance of his theory by the scientific community, in 1978 he was rewarded with the Nobel Prize for Chemistry, for what is now known as the chemiosmotic theory of the synthesis of ATP.

In outline, as reducing equivalents (or hydrogen atoms) are transferred through the enzymes of the electron transport chain towards their ultimate meeting with O_2, hydrogen ions (H^+) are pumped from the matrix across the inner mitochondrial membrane, and accumulate in the space between the inner and outer membranes, making a gradient of electrochemical potential (i.e. there is a build up of electrically charged particles). This process requires energy, which comes from the oxidation of the hydrogen atoms that have come from the citric acid cycle. The mitochondrial matrix, which has lost H^+ ions, ends up negatively charged with respect to the inner-membrane space, which becomes positively charged because it has gained H^+ ions. The voltage across the narrow inner membrane is about 200 millivolts. When these hydrogen ions flow back 'down' their gradient, energy will be liberated. This happens within an enzyme that is embedded in the inner mitochondrial

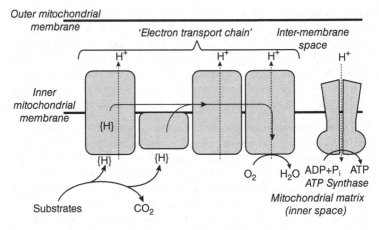

Figure 5.6 Oxidative phosphorylation: the synthesis of ATP (called phosphorylation) using energy derived from oxidation of nutrients (delivered to the system as 'reducing equivalents', or hydrogen atoms, shown as {H}). The grey shapes represent different enzymes making up the complex called the electron transport chain, and ATP synthase, the enzyme that makes ATP from ADP and P_i.

membrane called ATP synthase (because it makes – synthesises – ATP). ATP synthase is a complex enzyme, consisting of several separate proteins. It sits in the inner membrane of the mitochondrion, and as H^+ ions travel through a central channel, the inner part of the enzyme rotates, like a propeller, making ATP. You can see schematic videos online. This is illustrated in Figure 5.6. The workings of ATP synthase were investigated by several scientists using a variety of techniques before this final model was arrived at, and led to a Nobel Prize in Chemistry awarded in 1997 to Paul Boyer of the University of California and John Walker of the UK Medical Research Council's Laboratory of Molecular Biology in Cambridge (they shared the prize with the Danish scientist Jens Skou, who discovered an enzyme that uses ATP to move ions – in this case, sodium and potassium ions – across cell membranes, one of the big users of ATP, especially in nerve cells). The electron transport chain and ATP synthase are clustered together in the inner mitochondrial membrane.

So now we have seen how sugars, fats, some amino acids, and alcohol are broken down step-wise. Initially the result is a compound with two carbon atoms, acetic acid, in the form of acetyl-CoA. Acetyl-CoA is then oxidised, resulting in the loss of carbon dioxide, in the citric acid cycle. The hydrogen atoms that it loses are transferred to the electron transport chain, and as they combine with oxygen, the energy released is used to pump hydrogen ions, H^+, into the space between the two mitochondrial membranes. Finally, H^+ ions move back into the mitochondrial matrix through the enzyme ATP synthase, resulting in the synthesis of the energy-carrying molecule ATP.

One Glucose or Amino Acid Molecule Makes a Lot of ATP: Fatty Acids Even More

As we shall see shortly, there are uncertainties about the exact balance between hydrogen atoms transferred to the electron transport chain and molecules of ATP synthesised. However, taking typical values for this, the oxidation of one molecule of acetyl-CoA generates about 10 molecules of ATP.

If we consider the complete breakdown and oxidation of glucose, then we saw earlier that two molecules of ATP are generated by substrate-level phosphorylation before the glucose (as pyruvic acid) enters the mitochondrion. There are also some hydrogen atoms released onto the carrier NAD. Once pyruvate is inside the mitochondrion, it is acted upon by pyruvate dehydrogenase, to make acetyl-CoA, and this generates further hydrogen atoms, and so ATP. In all, one molecule of glucose leads to synthesis of about 32 molecules of ATP (older textbooks quote values of up to 38 molecules of ATP, but ideas have changed, partly because of more detailed understanding of the action of ATP synthase). Complete oxidation of glucose clearly yields much more energy (ATP) than does the first part of its breakdown in the cytoplasm. That will be highly relevant when we consider the need for energy during exercise. Similar figures would apply to many amino acids whose breakdown leads to formation of acetyl-CoA.

If we consider the oxidation of fatty acids, then the yield is even greater: oxidation of one molecule of palmitic acid, for example (saturated, 16 carbon atoms), yields something like 104 molecules of ATP (again, older textbooks may quote up to 129).

It is interesting to see just how much 'energy' has been trapped in ATP by these pathways. One molecule of ATP splitting into ADP and phosphate liberates energy. The amount of energy liberated, though, depends on the concentrations of the compounds involved, and other conditions, so is difficult to estimate in a cell, but a value of about 50 kJ per mole of ATP might be typical. (One mole is the molecular mass of ATP – that is, the mass of one molecule compared with a hydrogen atom, expressed in grams, in this case 507.) If we say that one molecule of glucose leads to 32 molecules of ATP, then, with glucose having a molecular mass of 180, we can calculate that each gram of glucose leads to about 9 kJ of energy trapped in ATP. If we were simply to burn the glucose, then each gram would liberate about 17 kJ. So, very approximately, half the chemical energy in the glucose molecule has been saved for the cell to use in the form of ATP. The rest must have been lost as heat. On the other hand, had the glucose been simply burned, all would have been lost as heat.

A Further Uncertainty in ATP Yields

No biological membrane is fully efficient as a barrier. All are to some extent leaky. The mechanism I have described for making ATP, whereby hydrogen ions (H^+) accumulate between the mitochondrial membranes, is no exception. There is evidence for some 'leakiness' of the inner mitochondrial membrane. This means that for each molecule of glucose, fatty acid, or amino acid oxidised, a variable amount of energy may be lost as heat and not stored as ATP. Indeed, there is a biological mechanism that makes direct use of this phenomenon – generation of heat by the tissue called brown fat. There are certain poisons that make the inner mitochondrial membrane leaky – one is called 2,4 dinitrophenol (often abbreviated DNP). A derivative of this material, 2,4-dichlorophenoxyacetic acid, is used as a herbicide – you can buy it for use in your garden under the general name 'brushwood killer'. But unfortunately it kills insects and other garden life also. Because of its property of making the inner mitochondrial membrane leaky, it is said to 'uncouple' the electron transport chain: reducing equivalents no longer generate ATP. Instead, energy is lost as heat. This sounds like a treatment that means nutrients are used and heat given off, not stored – the cure for obesity, perhaps. But be warned: people have tried this, and most have died. It is extremely toxic to humans. Perhaps we learn something from this: the systems we have to conserve energy have evolved over countless millennia, and we mess with them at our peril.

With the knowledge gained so far about metabolic fuel stores, metabolic pathways, how ATP is made, and how information is communicated, we can now have a look at what goes on inside us during normal daily life.

6 Metabolism in Daily Life

How We Study Human Metabolism

If your doctor wishes to assess the state of your metabolism, it is most likely she or he will start by taking a blood sample and sending it to a laboratory where the concentrations of various compounds can be measured.

This is extremely useful for the clinician. For instance, suppose the concentration of glucose in your blood turns out to be 10 mmol/l (see Box 4.1 for explanation of these units), when the normal concentration is around 5 mmol/l, then clearly there is a problem with your glucose metabolism.

But it does not tell us the nature of this problem. Suppose we notice there are more cars than usual on the main road near our house. Is that because there's a football match on, and more people than usual are out driving? Or does it tell us there are roadworks causing a blockage somewhere? To put that in metabolic terms, if a doctor were to find that a patient had an elevated concentration of glucose, is it that the liver is producing glucose too fast, or that the tissues that use glucose, such as muscles, aren't working well? For that, one needs a more dynamic approach.

There have been many developments in the study of human intermediary metabolism from the mid-twentieth century onwards. Rudolf Schoenheimer was yet another German biochemist who moved abroad to escape from the Nazi regime. He moved to Columbia University in New York and collaborated with other scientists there to pioneer the use of isotopes to study metabolism. The atoms of most elements can exist in different forms – differing numbers of neutrons in the nucleus give the atoms different masses, but the chemical properties, which depend on the numbers of charged protons and electrons, are unchanged. An example is hydrogen. Normally the nucleus of the hydrogen atom consists of just one proton (a positively charged particle), and is matched by one electron (negatively charged) circulating around it. This atom is conventionally thought of as having a mass of 1. But there is another form of hydrogen, in which a neutron is also present in the nucleus. The neutron and the proton have equal masses, so the mass of this atom is 2 (electrons are so small they make almost no difference). This is called an isotope of hydrogen. It can be written ^2H (not to be confused with H_2, which means a molecule containing two atoms of hydrogen). It has the name deuterium. It occurs naturally and accounts for approximately 0.02% of naturally occurring hydrogen (e.g. in water). The chemical properties of ^1H (normal hydrogen) and ^2H are virtually indistinguishable.

It is possible to make pure deuterium, and from that to make chemicals that contain it: an example would be glucose ($C_6H_{12}O_6$), in which one – or more – of the hydrogen atoms can be substituted with deuterium. A quick online search tells me that the Canadian company C/D/N Isotopes can supply me with 1 gram of 'D-Glucose-6,6-d_2' – meaning glucose in which the two hydrogen atoms attached to carbon no. 6 (see Figure 2.1) are replaced with deuterium (d in their nomenclature). This will behave in the body just like any other molecule of glucose, but with the important difference that the fate of the deuterium atoms can be followed. This glucose with deuterium would typically be called a 'tracer', as it is used to trace molecules through metabolic pathways, and we would call molecules containing the deuterium 'labelled'. For instance, the question might be: can glucose be converted into fatty acids? Some of the deuterium-labelled glucose might be injected into a vein of a volunteer (in a suitably sterile form), or the volunteer might drink it in a solution. Then at some point a blood sample could be taken, and the fatty acids separated out using solvents. Most of these fatty acids won't contain any deuterium, but some will. They need to be separated out from the 'unlabelled' fatty acids, when the only difference is in the mass of their molecules. This is done in a mass spectrometer – an instrument that separates compounds according to their molecular mass. So, for instance, it would be possible to look at different conditions (e.g. different diets, or to compare people with diabetes with non-diabetic people) to see what influences the appearance of the 'label' (deuterium) from glucose in the fatty acids.

Schoenheimer and his colleagues looked at fatty acids: they were able to show for the first time in people that fatty acids could be converted into one another. For instance, they showed that when deuterium-labelled stearic acid (saturated, like palmitic acid, but with 18 carbon atoms) was given to volunteers, the deuterium would appear in oleic acid (18 carbon atoms, monounsaturated) – this is the process called desaturation that I mentioned in Chapter 3. Schoenheimer was also interested in protein metabolism, and he used the nitrogen isotope ^{15}N, which is heavier than the normal ^{14}N, to label amino acids and follow their fate.

^{2}H (deuterium) and ^{15}N, and also ^{13}C, are stable atoms – they do not decay. They are called stable isotopes. A very similar technique uses isotopes that are not stable, and decay spontaneously – these are radioactive isotopes, for instance ^{3}H (known as tritium) and ^{14}C. Radioactive isotopes are easier to detect than stable isotopes – the radioactivity can be measured easily using an instrument like a Geiger counter, without the use of the mass spectrometer. But, of course, for human investigations, they pose some safety issues (not insurmountable, but needing careful control).

These isotopic tracers, as they are usually called, can be used to measure the turnover of metabolites in the bloodstream – even in tissues, if it's possible to sample the tissue concerned. (It's unusual to sample from a human liver for experimental purposes, although it has been done, as I mentioned in Chapter 2. Taking a small sample of muscle, usually from the leg, is fairly routine, using a special needle with a hollow core, under local anaesthetic. Taking a sample of fat is even easier: many volunteers urge us to take more.) If the isotopic tracer is pumped slowly into a vein, for instance, then its resulting concentration amongst the molecules it is tracing (for instance, the ratio of deuterium-labelled glucose to unlabelled glucose) will give the experimenter a measure of how fast the substance in the blood is turning over. This technique is regularly employed by researchers to study glucose, fatty acid, and amino acid metabolism.

Again, the field develops fast and now there is a range of new techniques based around newer imaging methods. Positron emission tomography (PET) uses very short-lived highly radioactive tracers – for instance, glucose labelled with a radioactive fluorine atom, which behaves metabolically like normal glucose – and these can be 'seen' from outside the body with a specialised camera. This technique is now widely used in diagnosis of tumours, since tumour cells have a high rate of glucose metabolism, so 'hot spots' of tracer will indicate where these are.

Daily Life as Opposed to Acute Stress

As I have mentioned, the first part of my career was spent studying patients who were acutely ill. Later, I became more interested in understanding how humans metabolise fat from the diet. Much of this work consisted of studying healthy volunteers, or patients with diabetes, for instance, who would arrive in the laboratory in the morning having fasted since the previous evening. We would then feed the volunteers a test meal, and follow their metabolism over the next few hours. In some experiments we would give them another meal after a suitable interval. That research was, in outline, very simple, although we were looking at metabolic pathways that had not been much explored in humans. But they were very revealing to me, given that I had worked for the previous 10 years with acutely ill patients with all sorts of problems, whose metabolism was dominated by a big stress response, with adrenaline, nor-adrenaline (from the sympathetic nervous system), and other stress hormones like cortisol playing a big role. Now I began to see how metabolism worked in normal daily life. This wasn't novel research (aside from the particular pathways we were studying), and what we found would not have surprised earlier generations of metabolic scientists: but, as I say, they were revealing for me, and formed the basis of a new way for me to look at how all of metabolism is integrated in the body. In this chapter I will try to share those insights with you.

Before Breakfast: Glucose Metabolism

The state of the body before breakfast, described as 'overnight fasted' or as 'postabsorptive' (meaning that all the nutrients from the last evening's meal have been absorbed from the intestine into the bloodstream), is taken in many metabolic experiments as a starting point. It is often thought of as a relatively stable state, although careful examination of people in this state, who continue to fast, show that it's just a point in a changing metabolic situation – as the body begins to assume no food is coming, and adapt to starvation. Nevertheless, it is at least a state that is fairly readily standardised.

The glucose concentration in blood will be around 4.5–5 mmol/l. It will be fairly steady, but that does not mean that the glucose is static: glucose will be used continuously (e.g. by the brain) and replaced, by glucose coming from the liver. In round figures, a little over 100 mg glucose will be leaving the bloodstream, and an equal amount replacing it, every minute – between 6 and 8 g every hour. There are about 4.5 g of glucose present in our blood (and maybe twice that amount in other fluid in the body – say 12–14 g in total), so the glucose in the blood turns over completely every 30–40 minutes. All the free glucose (that is, not combined in glycogen) will turn over every couple of hours.

Where does this glucose come from? Almost entirely the liver (since there is none coming from the intestine). It is coming approximately half from the breakdown (mobilisation) of the liver's glycogen store, and about half from the pathway of gluconeogenesis (making new glucose from other metabolites). These proportions are undoubtedly changing at this stage – the longer the fast continues, the more gluconeogenesis will contribute.

And where does the glucose from the blood go to? In round figures, the brain uses about 80 mg/min (of the approximately 130 mg/min total), and the rest is used by a variety of tissues including muscles, kidneys, blood cells, and fat cells.

There is a mechanism in operation here to conserve glucose. Glucose is precious. If we don't get it from what we eat, it must be made. The major source for making completely new glucose is amino acids. And – if we are not eating protein – using amino acids means breaking down the body's proteins. That is something that our bodies only do when nothing else is available, as loss of protein means loss of some function.

In Chapter 3, we looked at the process of breakdown of glucose ($C_6H_{12}O_6$), through the pathway of glycolysis, to make pyruvic acid ($C_3H_4O_3$). In some tissues, this pyruvate does not enter the citric acid cycle for complete combustion. Indeed, in some tissues that pathway does not exist – in others, it may not be very active, perhaps because oxygen supply is not adequate. The enzymes of the citric acid cycle are present in the mitochondria within cells, as we saw in Chapter 5. Red blood cells do not have mitochondria. So they cannot use fatty acids for energy (as that process requires the citric acid cycle). They can only generate energy (i.e. make ATP) by breaking down glucose to pyruvic acid (by substrate-level phosphorylation, as described in Chapter 5). The inner part of the kidney, called the medulla, has a rather poor blood supply and hence not much oxygen, and so mostly does the same. Under many conditions, this is also true of muscles. If pyruvate isn't broken down

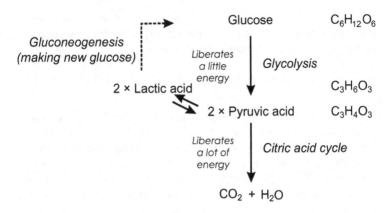

Figure 6.1 Steps in the breakdown of glucose.
All cells can metabolise glucose to pyruvic acid by the pathway called glycolysis. This liberates a little energy. Many cells, given adequate oxygen supply, can then oxidise the pyruvic acid completely to carbon dioxide (CO_2) and water (H_2O) in the citric acid cycle, liberating a lot of energy for use by the cell. But in cells that do not have this capacity, pyruvic acid is converted to lactic acid. If you compare the formula for lactic acid with that of glucose, you will see that it is exactly half a glucose molecule. In Figure 6.2 we will see that, in the liver, lactic acid can be converted back into glucose, so completing a cycle (pathway called gluconeogenesis, broken line).

further in the citric acid cycle (ultimately to CO_2 and water), it is converted to lactic acid. Lactic acid is $C_3H_6O_3$, and if you compare with glucose ($C_6H_{12}O_6$), you'll see it's exactly half a glucose molecule. This is the role of lactic acid – it is a breakdown product of glucose when pyruvate can't be metabolised further by combining with oxygen. Effectively the glucose molecule is split in half, although this occurs, as in all metabolic pathways, through multiple small steps. Some energy is released in the formation of lactic acid from glucose, although much less than if the pyruvic acid were to be oxidised in the citric acid cycle (Figure 6.1).

So, in tissues that do not have the capacity to further break down pyruvic acid, glucose is converted to lactic acid. In the process, some energy is liberated and can be used by the cell. But the big advantage to the organism is that the glucose is not lost forever. Lactic acid can be released into the bloodstream and carried back to the liver where, under these conditions, it is the major starting material for the pathway of gluconeogenesis – making new glucose. This pathway requires input of some energy – that's inevitable, given that energy was released in the production of lactic acid from glucose. But in the liver, this energy might be provided from various sources, including breakdown of fatty acids. Therefore tissues such as red blood cells, which cannot themselves derive energy other than by conversion of glucose to lactic acid, ultimately get their energy from fat. That is not often appreciated, even by biochemistry students, and has resulted in many puzzled looks when I have said it. In contrast, if pyruvic acid enters the citric acid cycle, it is broken down irreversibly (to CO_2 and H_2O), so losing glucose from the body.

This, then, is another metabolic cycle: the interconversion of glucose and lactic acid. It was discovered by a wife and husband team, Gerty and Carl Cori. In what seems like a common theme amongst Nobel Prize-winning metabolic biochemists of the early and mid-twentieth century, Gerty and Carl began their studies in Prague, continued their research in Vienna, and then were persuaded to move to the US by increasing antisemitism. Their important work on carbohydrate metabolism was done at what is now the Roswell Park Cancer Institute in Buffalo, New York. There they investigated glycogen breakdown, and discovered the cycle that is named after them, for which they jointly received the Nobel Prize in Physiology or Medicine in 1947, along with the Argentinian physiologist Bernardo Houssay, for his work on hormones and glucose metabolism.

This is an opportunity to say something more about glycogen in muscle. I mentioned in Chapter 2 that muscle glycogen, when broken down, cannot lead directly to the release of glucose into the bloodstream – only liver can do that. The reason is that the liver has an enzyme called enzyme glucose-6-phosphatase, which releases glucose from the intermediate called glucose 6-phosphate. (Glucose 6-phosphate is formed from glycogen breakdown, but it is also the starting point for glycogen synthesis, and for glucose breakdown in the pathway of glycolysis. It is a key interchange in the various routes for the metabolism of glucose.) So instead, in muscle, glycogen breakdown can lead to glucose molecules (in the form of glucose 6-phosphate) entering the pathway of glycolysis, with formation of lactic acid: that lactic acid can then travel to the liver to be made into glucose. So, whilst muscle glycogen cannot contribute directly to glucose in the blood, it can do so indirectly through this pathway described by the Coris (Figure 6.2).

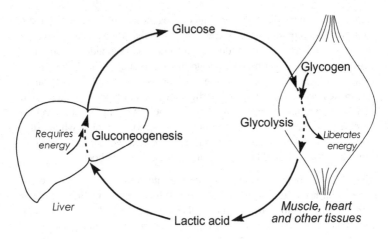

Figure 6.2 The Cori cycle.

Before Breakfast: Fat Metabolism

Glucose is important at this early stage of fasting, and as we have seen keeps vital organs such as the brain supplied with fuel. However, in the body as a whole, glucose is typically only supplying around one third of energy requirements after an overnight fast. The rest is mainly supplied by fat, with some contribution from amino acids.

As we have seen, use of fat for energy involves the triacylglycerol in our fat cells being broken down to liberate fatty acids, which can travel through the bloodstream to tissues such as heart and muscle, where they supply most of the energy requirements in this overnight-fasted state. The fat cells, or adipocytes, are not spread randomly around the body but are collected together in areas that are known as fat (or adipose) depots. Caroline Pond, working at the UK's Open University, has studied these fat depots: she has dissected many species, from polar bears and tigers, to small mammals brought to her laboratory as road kill. Some fat depots are common to all mammals but the 'tummy fat', strictly called the subcutaneous anterior abdominal fat depot (or 'paunch' in Caroline's terminology), is only found to any great extent in humans and other primates. As well as adipocytes, these fat depots contain other cell types, including stem cells called preadipocytes that can differentiate into new adipocytes. There are also supporting cells, and – as Caroline Pond has shown – immune cells such as those in lymph nodes embedded in the adipose tissue, that may benefit from the presence of readily available fatty acids.

Fatty acids can be used as a fuel only by tissues that can use oxygen and finally break them down in the citric acid cycle. (There is no equivalent to the 'glycolysis' pathway for fatty acids.) In the overnight-fasted state the main consumers of fatty acids will be the liver (as we have seen, fatty acids can supply the energy needed to make glucose in the liver), heart, muscles, and the outer part of the kidneys, the cortex. The kidney cortex has a good blood supply and therefore plenty of oxygen delivery, unlike the central part, or medulla, of the kidneys which has a poor blood supply in relation to meta-bolic needs and mainly uses glucose, delivering back lactic acid. The brain cannot use fatty acids directly as fuel – this has repercussions for metabolism during starvation that we shall look at in Chapter 7.

Amino Acids after Fasting Overnight

The regulation of amino acid and protein metabolism has some similarities with carbohydrate and fat, but also many differences.

Our tissues are largely made of proteins (with a lot of water, and variable amounts of fat depending on the tissue). The individual types of protein turn over at different rates – that is, they are broken down to amino acids, and resynthesised. Some turn over rapidly, others more slowly. On average around 3% of the body's proteins are replaced each day. For most people, the total amount of protein in the body will remain steady from day to day, but that hides some variation during the day. Just like carbohydrate and fat, protein synthesis is regulated by insulin, although not to the same rapid extent. There is some overall breakdown of protein in the fasting state, and more synthesis after meals. A bigger driver of protein synthesis, especially in muscle, is physical activity – as in 'body building'. The use of amino acids as an energy source must reflect their availability, from a net breakdown of protein or, after meals, as we shall see, from what we eat.

So, in typical daily life, after an overnight fast there is some net breakdown of protein, and amino acids are used as an energy source. A round figure would be that oxidation of amino acids contributes 10–15% of energy production after fasting overnight. This will occur in many tissues but predominantly muscles (not least because they have the largest amount of protein) and liver.

We saw in the previous chapter that, unlike carbohydrates and fats, amino acids cannot be fully oxidised to CO_2 and water, since they also (by definition) contain atoms of nitrogen (N); this is transferred into the relatively non-toxic compound urea in the liver and excreted in the urine.

The Human Gut (Gastrointestinal Tract)

It is with the arrival of a meal that we see the wonders of human metabolism and how it is integrated throughout the body. We will start with a quick look at what goes on in the gut, or gastrointestinal tract, illustrated in Figure 6.3.

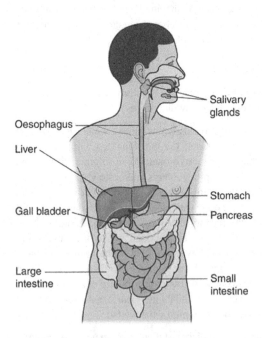

Figure 6.3   The human gastrointestinal (digestive) tract.

The process we call digestion is a breakdown of food: mechanical break-down, using our teeth and then the churning action of the stomach, into finer and finer particles, and chemical breakdown, so that the polymers – starch, fats, proteins – are broken down into their smaller components (sugars, fatty acids, amino acids). These can then be absorbed through the wall of the intestine into the bloodstream. Some of this digestion occurs in the mouth and in the stomach, but more follows as the food enters the small intestine, the first 3–4 metres after the stomach. Most digestion and absorption is completed as food passes through the small intestine. The large intestine, or colon, is the final part of the tract, about 1.5 metres in length, from the end of the small intestine (the part called the ileum) to the anus. Any food materials not digested in the small intestine arrive here and are acted upon by microorganisms that live in the colon. We will touch on that again later.

Toast for Breakfast

Breakfast may contain a reasonable amount of carbohydrate – toast or cereals, for instance. Starch digestion begins in the mouth as the food is chewed, by the action of the enzyme amylase in saliva. (Amylase is a general term for an enzyme that acts on starch to break off individual glucose units. Starch consists of two components: amylose and amylopectin. These enzymes involved in digestion are called α-amylases as they act on bonds between glucose molecules in the so-called α-configuration, as they are in starch. In cellulose, found in plant cell walls, the glucose units are β-linked, and our enzymes cannot break these bonds. They may be broken by bacterial enzymes in the colon.) This digestion continues as the food reaches the stomach, although the acid produced by the stomach walls then stops it, as the amylase enzyme can't function in acid conditions. Once the food reaches the small intestine, it meets the digestive juices produced by the pancreas – these include a bicarbonate-rich solution that neutralises the stomach acid (so that digestive enzymes can work more readily), and another α-amylase, pancreatic amylase, which largely breaks down the starch to di- and mono-saccharides. Finally, there are some enzymes produced by the cells of the small intestine themselves which break down any remaining disaccharides to release the monosaccharides (mainly glucose and fructose from sucrose, and galactose from the milk sugar lactose). These are taken up, through the cells that line the small intestine, and into the bloodstream.

I noted before that cell membranes are made of lipids, and water-soluble molecules like sugars cannot easily cross them. The intestinal cells make proteins that form specific channels for glucose and other sugars to cross (both into the cell, from the intestine, and out from the cell, into the blood). These proteins belong to the large family of glucose transporters. Some, such as those in the small intestine responsible for taking up glucose into the cells, use energy, so that the glucose can be moved into a region of higher concentration, something that would not happen by itself. We can imagine that, towards the end of absorbing the glucose from a meal, the concentration inside the intestine is now quite low, but there is plenty within the cells, and in the blood beyond, so these energy-requiring channels allow those last bits of glucose to be taken up and not lost. The transporters allowing glucose to enter the blood from the intestinal cells are different: they are proteins making glucose-shaped pores in the membrane, and glucose will travel through from a higher concentration in the cell to a lower concentration in the blood, without input of energy. They belong to the family known as GLUTs (glucose transporters).

The blood supply to the small intestine is rich, and variable in time. It increases after a meal, so there is plenty of blood to take away the products of digestion. The veins that drain the blood away from the small intestine merge and go straight to the liver in the big vessel called the hepatic portal vein. So the products of starch digestion reach the liver before they get to other tissues. This makes good sense, as the liver is the main site where spare glucose can be stored, as glycogen.

So now the liver needs to stop what it is doing – breaking down glycogen, making new glucose – and begin to store the spare glucose. How does it know to do this? The answer is largely through insulin.

Some glucose will travel straight through the liver, and, via the large veins that drain the liver, the hepatic veins, will reach the general circulation (bloodstream). The concentration of glucose in the blood, as we have seen, is typically 4.5–5 mmol/l after an overnight fast. Now it will begin to rise. This blood is reaching all organs, including the pancreas and, within the pancreas, the islets of Langerhans. Within the β-cells of these islets, glucose metabolism will increase, and this is a signal for the β-cells to release more insulin. (Insulin release will have been at a low level during the overnight fast.) This insulin is released into the veins that drain the islets, and these run, not into the general circulation, but straight into the hepatic portal vein, so, like the products of starch digestion, reaching the liver. Here the insulin acts on insulin receptors in the liver cells and leads to changes in enzyme activity, including switching off glycogen phosphorylase (breaking down glycogen) and activation of glycogen synthase (making new glycogen). In addition, the pathway of gluconeogenesis (making new glucose) is suppressed. So the liver cells begin to take in glucose, to store some as glycogen, and to use glucose as a fuel.

Insulin is also a signal to other tissues to use glucose. In muscles, there are changes very like those in liver: glycogen breakdown ceases, glycogen synthesis is turned on, and glucose is used as a fuel. (Muscles don't have the pathway of gluconeogenesis for making new glucose.) In muscle cells there is a clever mechanism to aid these changes. Muscles have a particular form of the glucose transporter protein (that enables glucose to cross cell membranes) called GLUT4 (GLUT denotes a member of the family of transporters that allow glucose through without using energy). Muscle cells always have plenty of GLUT4, but in the absence of an insulin signal, this is tucked away inside the cells. When the insulin signal is sensed, GLUT4 moves to the cell membrane to allow glucose to enter. GLUT4 is known as the insulin-regulated glucose transporter.

In fat cells (adipocytes) something similar happens: fat cells also have GLUT4 and take up more glucose when insulin signals them to do so. They use glucose for energy and for dealing with fatty acids.

The brain, on the other hand, does not have GLUT4; it has other glucose transporters that allow glucose to be taken up at a fairly constant rate whatever the glucose concentration in blood (except when it is particularly low). The brain goes on using glucose at a virtually constant rate whatever we might have eaten. This makes good sense – we would not want to be super-intelligent only after eating a meal.

Before leaving this section, I will just say something about hormones and the metabolism they control with some data from our own experiments. Healthy volunteers came into our laboratory, having fasted overnight. We gave them a breakfast containing carbohydrates, fats, and proteins in roughly the proportions they occur in the average UK diet. We found that both glucose and insulin concentrations in the blood reached a peak at 1 hour after eating the meal. Table 6.1 shows the average values.

	Before breakfast	60 minutes later	% increase
Glucose (mmol/l)	5.0	8.2	65%
Insulin (pmol/l)	38	546	1 340%

Note that insulin goes through a much greater 'excursion' in relative terms (i.e. in relation to its own baseline) than does glucose: more than 1 000% compared with less than 100%. This is typical where one variable is controlling another. An analogy would be the electric current through a heating element keeping a water bath at an almost constant temperature. A thermostat will switch on the current when the water temperature drops below a certain threshold, and turn it off when the water temperature reaches a point just above that desired. The electric current will vary between zero and whatever is needed, whereas the water temperature may only vary by a few per cent either side of the 'set-point'. So we can be sure that insulin is there to regulate the glucose concentration in blood.

Table 6.1   Glucose and insulin concentrations in volunteers before and 1 hour after a test meal

Butter on the Toast

Now we can explore what happens to fat metabolism after breakfast. The breakfast might contain fat in butter on the toast, or perhaps rather more fat in a bacon and egg sandwich. But even if there is no fat, there will be changes in fat metabolism as the body changes to storage mode.

The same principles of digestion that we have already explored with carbohydrates apply to fat. Here the digestion involves breaking up the fat into the smallest possible droplets, so that enzymes can act on as much surface area as possible. The enzymes break down the triacylglycerols, the form in which most dietary fat exists. These enzymes belong to the general group known as lipases: enzymes that act on lipids (fat). In rodents, there is – like salivary amylase – a lipase secreted in the mouth, and for many years it was assumed that humans had the same. But we don't – we have a related lipase produced in the stomach. This enzyme, unlike salivary amylase, is active even in the acidic environment of the stomach, and begins the process of digesting the fat. Most of the digestion, however, takes place in the small intestine, brought about by a pancreatic enzyme, pancreatic lipase.

Large droplets of fat need to be made smaller – dispersed into microscopic droplets in the process called emulsification. This is exactly the same process as cleaning grease with soap, as we saw in Chapter 2. In the intestine, it is brought about by some powerful detergents that are produced by the liver, called bile salts. The bile salts are derived from cholesterol in the liver – in fact, production of bile salts is one of the few mechanisms the body has for getting rid of excess cholesterol. They are stored in the gall bladder, and then released into the small intestine when fat arrives there. The pancreatic digestive juices also arrive at just the required time.

How do the gall bladder and the pancreas know when to release their contents into the small intestine? Once again, hormones are involved. The stomach itself, and the walls of the small intestine, contain cells that secrete hormones – so-called entero-endocrine cells. These hormones were amongst the earliest discovered. The first hormone to be discovered was secretin, a small protein hormone (it has 27 amino acids) that is produced by cells in the small intestinal wall when the acidic mixture from the stomach arrives. Secretin was identified by the British physiologists William Bayliss and Ernest Starling in 1902. (Starling also introduced the word 'hormone'.) Secretin signals to the pancreas to secrete its bicarbonate-rich fluid to neutralise the stomach acid. Another hormone released at the same time has the name cholecystokinin, CCK. That name refers to the fat that CCK signals to the gall bladder to contract and release its bile into the intestine. It also signals to the pancreas to release its digestive enzymes – originally this was thought to be the role of a separate hormone, called pancreozymin, before it was discovered that pancreozymin and CCK are one and the same.

Now the pancreatic lipase can begin seriously to attack the fat that remains, acting over a large surface area. It liberates fatty acids from the triacylglycerols. But the triacylglycerols are not entirely hydrolysed – broken down – to fatty acids and glycerol. Some triacylglycerols have one fatty acid removed, so they become diacylglycerols, and then fatty acids and diacylglycerols, and probably some monoacylglycerols, are absorbed into the intestinal cells. (Monoacylglycerol molecules, with one water-fearing fatty acid chain and several water-loving groups, are excellent emulsifying agents, and help the process of digestion as they are produced. Monoacylglycerols are widely used as emulsifying agents in the catering industry.)

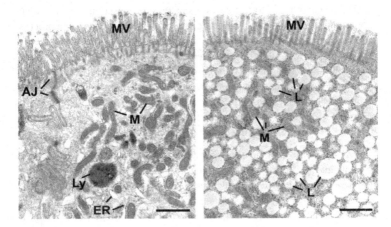

Figure 6.4   Intestinal cells with fat.
The pictures show intestinal cells as seen under high magnification in the electron microscope. On the left is a sample taken after the patient had fasted overnight. On the right is a sample taken a few hours after the patient drank 50 g of fat in the form of a fatty drink. 'MV' are the microvilli – projections from an intestinal cell, into the intestine, that increase the surface area for absorbing nutrients. 'M' are the mitochondria, structures within the cell responsible for oxidation of substrates (see Chapter 5). 'L' on the right-hand picture are lipid droplets, looking like white circles, accumulating in the intestinal cell.

The intestinal cells may become full of fat droplets as the mono- and di-acylglycerols and the fatty acids are recombined into triacylglycerols. Dr Denise Robertson worked in my laboratory on fat digestion, with Derek Jewell, Professor of Gastroenterology in Oxford, and obtained samples of small intestinal wall from people after they had taken a fatty drink. These show clearly the accumulation of fat in the intestinal cells (Figure 6.4).

We saw briefly, in Chapter 2, how fat from the intestine, in the form of triacylglycerols, enters the bloodstream as a milk-like emulsion. (Figure 2.5 showed how the blood plasma will turn cloudy after a fatty meal.)

The fat within the emulsion droplets can find its way into a number of tissues, especially adipose tissue for fat storage: this process is itself stimulated by insulin. Muscles, including the heart muscle, can use the fat, although that

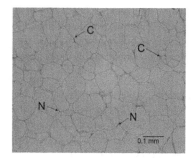

Figure 6.5 Human adipocytes (fat cells) under the microscope.
The picture shows a sample of fat taken from under the skin of the abdomen of a research volunteer. Each of the pale shapes is an individual fat cell. The cell membranes have been stained dark. 'C' represents a blood capillary (there are more capillaries, but they do not show up easily); 'N' is the nucleus (each fat cell has one but, again, they do not all show up clearly). The pale area within each cell is the droplet of fat (triacylglycerols) – there is very little else in each cell. They can be quite big – the little bar at the bottom right shows 0.1 mm.

process is not activated by insulin, so does not play a special role after a meal. The pathway for taking up this fat is complex (but interesting): indeed, it is one of the pathways that has been the focus of my career studying human fat metabolism. Adipocytes are amazingly specialised cells for storing fat, as you can see in Figure 6.5.

To make a parallel with glucose metabolism, we saw that insulin turns off glucose liberation from glycogen, and production of glucose from other sources, and at the same time stimulates the storage and utilisation of glucose. We have seen now that insulin promotes storage of fat in adipose tissue after a meal. Now we shall see that it also switches off fatty acid liberation (fat mobilisation).

Fat mobilisation is the process of liberation of fatty acids from the triacylglycerol stored in our fat cells. This process is brought about by enzymes that operate within the fat cells. As we have seen, the triacylglycerol molecule consists of three fatty acid molecules joined to one of glycerol. Enzymes remove these fatty acids one by one, so finally producing three fatty acids to be liberated into the plasma, and a molecule of glycerol. This is brought about by three distinct enzymes acting sequentially. After removal of one fatty acid, the remaining molecule is called a diacylglycerol (two fatty acids linked to glycerol), then it becomes a monoacylglycerol, before losing the last fatty acid. We met di- and mono-acylglycerols earlier, formed during the digestion of fat in the intestine.

Research on the middle of these three enzymes, acting on the diacylglycerols, has a long history. It is called hormone-sensitive lipase. Its name reflects the fact that it can be shown in the laboratory to be very rapidly activated by adrenaline. This is important in stress states, such as exercise, when we need to mobilise our fat stores to use as a fuel. But the main hormone regulating hormone-sensitive lipase in normal daily life is probably not adrenaline: it is insulin. When we have been fasting overnight, insulin concentrations in blood are low – the lowest they will be in a typical 24-hour period. Insulin very powerfully suppresses the activity of hormone-sensitive lipase. It does this by reducing the cellular concentration of cyclic AMP – we met cyclic AMP (cAMP) in the regulation of glycogen metabolism by hormones (see Figure 4.3). This is probably the metabolic process most sensitive to insulin in the human body – it responds to very small changes in insulin concentration. When insulin concentrations are low, before breakfast, fat mobilisation is going on at a good rate to supply fatty acids to other tissues, as we saw earlier. As soon as some glucose enters the circulation, and insulin begins to rise, fat mobilisation switches off. So, just as with glucose metabolism, the metabolic state changes from one of mobilisation of fuel stores to one of storage. It is important to note that the first enzyme in the process, called adipose tissue triacylglycerol lipase (ATGL), is also regulated by insulin, but not in such a direct manner.

So we see the importance of insulin in integrating the metabolic changes over a typical day. We mostly think of insulin as a hormone that regulates blood sugar (glucose). As we have seen, it is quite easy to measure the glucose concentration in blood, and has been for many years. In contrast, measurement of fatty acid concentrations requires more specialised techniques, and was never so readily available as glucose measurement. Vincent Marks at the University of Surrey, UK, is an expert on insulin (he is well known to the public not least for his role in investigating the use of insulin in murder cases). Vincent Marks has remarked that 'if only we could measure fatty acids as easily as we can measure glucose, we would think of diabetes as a disorder of fat metabolism'.

Add in Some Protein

Many breakfasts will also contain some protein – in dairy products, meat, or even in cereals. The same strategy applies to protein digestion. An enzyme secreted by the stomach, pepsin, starts the process of breaking apart the amino acids that make up proteins. (Its action is aided by the fact that the stomach acid will disrupt the folded structure of the protein – the process known as denaturation. This makes the bonds between amino acids more accessible.) Further digestion takes place in the small intestine, brought about by enzymes from the pancreas and those produced by the intestinal cells themselves. The products are individual amino acids, and some di- and tri-peptides (two or three amino acids joined), which can be absorbed into the intestinal cells, and thence enter the bloodstream, and, like glucose, they first pass through the liver, which will selectively remove some of the amino acids that it needs for its own purposes.

We have seen that muscle contains the largest amount of protein in the body, and there is strong evidence, based on feeding volunteers isotopically labelled amino acids and then taking small samples of muscle with a hollow needle, that insulin increases the synthesis of protein, so making a parallel with glucose and fat metabolism. So the body switches to a protein-building phase, although as noted earlier, muscle protein really needs the addition of physical activity to boost protein synthesis.

Unlike carbohydrate and fat, as we have seen before, there is no specific storage form of protein. The tissues will take the amino acids that they require to rebuild proteins lost during the overnight fast, but there is a long-standing observation that an excess of protein in a meal will be quickly oxidised, taking priority in the hierarchy of substrates to be used. Hans Krebs reviewed this old observation and showed how it is explained by the kinetic properties of the enzymes involved. The metabolic implication is that you can't build muscles just by eating a lot of protein – protein is necessary, but only adds muscle bulk if exercise provides the stimulus.

The mobilisation of fuel stores in the fasting state and rebuilding in the fed state is illustrated schematically in Figure 6.6.

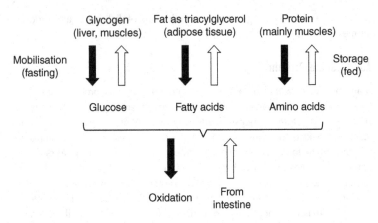

Figure 6.6 Integration of fuel mobilisation in the fasting state and rebuilding of stores in the fed state. Black arrows indicate mobilisation; white, storage. This integration is largely brought about by the hormone insulin.

The Colon and Human Metabolism

Materials that cannot be digested and absorbed in the small intestine arrive in the large intestine, or colon. This includes plant materials such as cellulose, for which we do not have digestive enzymes, and also some types of starch that form crystalline structures in food and hence cannot be reached by our digestive enzymes. Collectively all this material is called dietary fibre. Views of dietary fibre have changed considerably over recent years. At one time, material entering the colon was considered unwanted waste. In the late 1970s the British surgeon Denis Burkitt, already well known for describing the cancer called Burkitt's lymphoma, drew attention to the importance of adequate fibre in the diet for maintaining intestinal health. The view changed again from the 1990s onward, when the variety of microorganisms that inhabit the human colon was recognised. Each of us has a number of microorganisms, mainly bacteria, in our colon that is similar to the number of cells in the rest of our body. These microorganisms secrete enzymes that act upon the materials reaching the colon in a process called fermentation. It occurs in the virtual absence of oxygen, but results in the modification, and to some extent breakdown, of the material. Some of the products can be absorbed through the colon wall into the bloodstream and may contribute to, or otherwise affect, our metabolism.

A detailed description of the role on the intestinal microflora is beyond the scope of this book, but one group of products of fermentation is of interest. Some carbohydrate materials can be broken down to produce fatty acids with small numbers of carbon atoms, especially acetic acid (with two carbon atoms), propionic acid (with three), and butyric acid (with four). These small molecules evaporate easily ('volatility'), so these are known as the volatile (or short-chain) fatty acids. Butyric acid has a special role as a fuel for the cells lining the colon, the colonocytes, and may play a role in protecting against development of bowel cancer. Acetic and propionic acids may be taken up into the bloodstream and thus enter the metabolic pathways we have looked at: acetic acid can be converted into acetyl-CoA, propionic acid, after some metabolic modification, can enter the citric acid cycle or be converted to glucose. In this way, some of the energy in foodstuffs that might otherwise have been lost 'down the pan' is saved. Other mammals have evolved much more efficient means for doing just this. Cellulose in plants (such as grass) is a major fuel for ruminant animals, such as cows and sheep. These herbivores have a specialised intestinal tract with multiple stomachs, each containing a complement of microorganisms to help them digest these plant materials and harvest the energy contained within them.

Daily Metabolism and Energy Balance

We see, then, just how very dynamic human metabolism is even during a normal – but sedentary – day. Each of our major nutrients, carbohydrate, fat, and protein, is handled in its own way, but with the similarity that when there is an excess above immediate needs, it is channelled into storage, and then drawn from these stores as required (a little less clearly so for protein), and that much of the changing of metabolic state is signalled by the hormone insulin.

It will now be interesting to see what happens when these peaceful, well-fed days are interrupted, either by a lack of food, or by a sudden need to expend more energy during exercise.

7 Metabolism Is So Adaptable

Why Our Metabolism Needs to Be Adaptable

Our metabolism has by necessity to be very adaptable. It adapts during each day as we eat and exercise. It adapts if we change our habits – change our diet or change our lifestyle. It adapts as we age, from a very fat-based economy (milk) in our very early days, to whatever we might choose to eat as adults. The ability to conduct these adaptations has been shaped by our evolution. Famine has been an intermittent but powerful shaping force. The need to be able to exercise has always been important, from hunter-gatherer days through the development of agriculture, involving much manual labour: only in very recent years has it been possible for many people to lead lives that may involve little physical exertion each day amidst plentiful food.

There is a great contrast between starvation, when our metabolism slows down as the body attempts to conserve its remaining resources, and physical activity, when metabolism proceeds at a faster rate than at rest. Study of metabolism in both these fields has a long history.

Survival during Starvation, and Physical Activity, Both Need Cooperation between Tissues

If I take a cell from a volunteer, say a fat cell, a liver cell, or a muscle cell, and put it in a flask in the laboratory, and give it what it needs such as sugar, oxygen, and amino acids, it may or may not continue to live for some time. It is unlikely to last for more than a day or so. (Cells can be grown for much longer periods, in the technique known as cell culture, but usually they are specialised cells that are precursor – stem – cells, or they are more like tumour cells that are more immortal than most adult human cells.) And yet, humans deprived of food can last many weeks, even months. This is because the different organs in the body cooperate to maintain life.

Similar statements can be made about exercise. The muscles, as we have seen, hold some fuel reserves in the form of glycogen, and a small, variable amount of fat. But this would not be sufficient to last more than some minutes of intense exercise. Longer exercise than that requires fuels to be provided from other tissues – glucose from the liver, fat from fat stores especially. These need to be delivered through the bloodstream, as does the oxygen needed to oxidise them. Blood is also needed to take away the waste products, including lactic acid and carbon dioxide, and these need to be disposed of in other tissues. So exercise, like starvation, is not something that can occur in a single cell: both information and cooperation are needed.

Studies of Human Starvation

The metabolic changes that occur to enable the body to continue to live without food have been the subject of research for a very long time.

Francis Benedict, of the University of Connecticut, was a pioneer of 'human calorimetry' in the early twentieth century. He built a chamber in which someone could spend long periods, in which oxygen consumption and carbon dioxide production could be measured: similar to Lavoisier's measurements (Figure 1.1), but allowing the volunteer more freedom. Benedict wrote a long report on 'A study of prolonged fasting', published in 1915. In the introduction, he described earlier observations of volunteers fasting for periods of up to 40 days, several of these fasts being made by an Italian named Succi. However, Benedict did not consider that these studies were scientifically based, and wished to undertake his own observations. In the report he described his search for a suitable volunteer. It happened that Succi came to New York, and had a conversation with Benedict, but, Benedict noted, 'his age and his somewhat unreasonable demands for a large compensation made an arrangement with him undesirable'. He also ruled out a number of individuals who came forward, but of whom he considered 'a large majority ... were either sufferers or imagined that they were sufferers from "nervous disease" and were therefore pathologically or psychologically undesirable'. Benedict then received a letter from a Maltese lawyer, Agostino

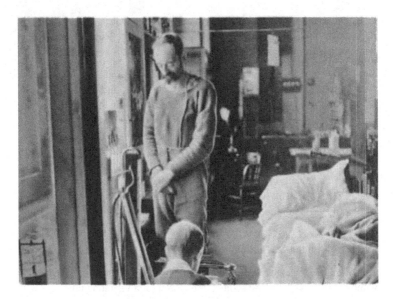

Figure 7.1   Levanzin being weighed on the 31st and last day of his fast.

Levanzin, who offered his services (Figure 7.1). Levanzin came to Boston to be briefed, the protocol was agreed, and once the experimental fast had begun, he wrote notes on his own life. He claimed to have previously fasted for 40 days for the sake of his health, and to have 'cured' a number of people of various ailments, including smallpox, by persuading them to fast for long periods.

Benedict studied Levanzin in detail over 31 days of fasting: Benedict had intended it to be 30 days, Levanzin claimed to be feeling fine and wanted to go on for 40 days, so they compromised on 31 as that broke the previous 'record of the longest controlled scientific fast ever made'. During this time, Levanzin's body weight fell from 60.6 kg to 47.4 kg (he started the fast in quite a thin state). Benedict noted that the rate of weight loss was greatest during the first few days, as water was lost from the body. Levanzin's urine was collected throughout, and amongst the measurements made was the total amount of nitrogen excreted in the urine: we will look more at the significance of this, but essentially it reflects breakdown of amino acids. This went from around 14 g/day before the fast, down to about 7 g/day at the end, reflecting a 'sparing' of amino acid breakdown: this is one of the most important adaptations to fasting, preserving the body's protein. Levanzin slept in the calorimeter. His oxygen consumption at night dropped from about 210–220 millilitres/minute (ml/min) at the beginning, to 160 ml/min at the end. This is another key adaptation: reduction in the total rate of metabolism, hence sparing the body's energy reserves. In terms of total heat produced, or energy expended, this translated to a fall from about 6.1 MJ/24 hours (1 500 kcal/24 hours) to 4.5 MJ/24 hours (1 100 kcal). There was an unpleasant end to this study. Levanzin became irritated after the end of the fast because Benedict required him to go into a hospital bed for a while for recuperation: Levanzin had been expecting some high-class convalescent home. Later, after his return to Malta, he made accusations that the experimenters had tried to poison him with sulphuric acid and, the *New York Times* reported, 'asserted that he had been squeezed like a lemon and then put out while he was weak and starving'.

A very well-known study on partial starvation was conducted by the American nutritionist Ancel Keys during the Second World War. Keys later became known for his work on cardiovascular disease, and his identification of saturated fats in the diet as a cause of elevated blood cholesterol concentration. Keys recognised that, as the war drew to a close, there would be an enormous need for scientific knowledge about how best to help those who had suffered malnutrition in its later years. He recruited a group of conscientious objectors at the University of Minnesota. Thirty-six of these men were studied over a period of 48 weeks, with 12 weeks of baseline study whilst receiving 13.4 MJ (3 200 kcal) daily, 24 weeks of semi-starvation, the men receiving food such that their body weight fell by 24% on average, and finally 12 weeks of rehabilitation on diets supplying different amounts of energy. The men were required to remain physically active by walking 22 miles each week. This was known as the Minnesota Experiment. Keys published the results in 1950 as a two-volume tome, *The Biology of Human Starvation*, with nearly 1 400 pages. Researchers today continue to work on the data it produced. Apart from the value of the results of the study, this report contained extensive reviews of the relevant literature.

The men rapidly lost fat from their bodies, so much so that they found sitting uncomfortable, and felt cold even in the summer. They described intense feelings of hunger – indeed, three men were excluded after cheating, and Keys excluded the data from another whose results he felt he could not trust. An important finding about the recovery period is that Keys realised that a very high energy intake was needed to reverse the effects of the semi-starvation phase: he noted that 'our experiments have shown that in an adult man no appreciable rehabilitation can take place on a diet of 8.4 MJ (2 000 kcal) a day. The proper level is more like 16.8 MJ (4 000 kcal) daily for some months. The character of the rehabilitation diet is important also, but unless calories are abundant, then extra proteins, vitamins and minerals are of little value'. (I have converted to MJ.)

Not all our knowledge of starvation comes from scientific experiments. Observations have been made on starvation during war – for instance, the Dutch famine of 1944–1945 when the Nazis stopped supply trains entering the Netherlands. Studies of the survivors of that period, and of their offspring, are still on-going. (They have revealed interesting effects of starvation on the 'epigenome' – the system whereby the DNA can be modified to change expression of certain genes.) And some people have starved themselves voluntarily. In 1980 and 1981, Irish republican prisoners in Northern Ireland began refusing food in the Irish hunger strikes, to back their demands to be treated as political prisoners rather than as criminals. In 1981, 10 of these prisoners, including their leader Bobby Sands, starved themselves to death. Tragic though this time was, there are some medical records that add to our understanding of what happens during starvation, and what determines the time someone can survive.

Our detailed, modern understanding of the metabolic changes in starvation comes from studies made in the 1960s, when physicians in Boston, US, treated a group of obese people by 'therapeutic starvation'. The patients were brought into hospital, and starved, other than water and vitamin and mineral supplements, for long periods. These people also volunteered to have various measurements made on them. Information from these observations has greatly improved our understanding of responses to starvation, although we should bear in mind the caveat that the subjects were people who were initially obese. George Cahill, a physician and scientist, was the lead investigator, and wrote many scientific papers on this topic.

Oliver Owen, a junior colleague of Cahill's and co-author on many of the papers, has written a personal account of the background to these experiments. It seems that before Cahill initiated these detailed studies, other obese patients had been 'fasted' for long periods, but allowed small amounts of carbohydrate. Owen describes an obese patient treated at the Johns Hopkins Hospital, Baltimore, who 'fasted' for 14 months: but Owen remembers the patient 'saying something like, "I need to drink a cola because my brain needs sugar".'

Metabolic Changes in Starvation: An Overview

A summary of key metabolic changes that occur during starvation is as follows. Whole-body metabolism, or energy expenditure, falls. Of course, people fasting usually become less active, but the fall is also seen in the resting metabolic rate, as measured at rest after fasting overnight – as we saw with Levanzin in Benedict's study. The fall in energy expenditure is more than would just be explained by the drop in body mass. This clearly reduces the need to draw on the body's fuel reserves. It is brought about mainly by a decrease in secretion of thyroid hormone, especially the active form called T_3. This fall in thyroid hormone secretion may be due, in turn, to lesser secretion of the hormone leptin from fat cells, as these cells sense a fuel deficit. Along with the reduction in whole-body metabolism, there is a sparing (reduction) of protein breakdown. This is often assessed as nitrogen excretion in the urine. When an amino acid is completely oxidised, its nitrogen is excreted, mainly in the form of urea (via the urea cycle in the liver), with some also as ammonia – the excretion of ammonia relative to urea increases as fasting progresses. The body's carbohydrate reserves, the glycogen stores, are quickly depleted. Liver glycogen, as we saw in Chapter 2, is depleted within 24 hours. There are not good data on muscle glycogen in human starvation, but judging from work in animals this might take a week or so. That was borne out in Benedict's study of Levanzin: he appeared to stop oxidising existing carbohydrate after about 1 week. (Remember that for the body to use *muscle* glycogen, it must be exported from the muscle, for instance as lactic acid, which can then be made into glucose in the liver.) Amino acid breakdown is, as just noted, reduced: specific mechanisms for this are not entirely clear although the reduction in whole-body metabolism will contribute. That leaves our fat stores as the main supplier of energy.

The observations that we have of death from starvation bear out the idea that essentially survival depends on the fat stores. These are gradually used up, and at the point that they are exhausted, then there is a rapid breakdown of protein, and death follows quickly. If we say (see Chapter 2) that the average amount of fat in the adult human body is around 25 kg, we can do a calculation. Metabolic rate falls – let's say (round figures) from 10 MJ/day (2 500 kcal/day) to maybe 7–8 MJ/day (1 700–1 900 kcal/day) (these are on the high side for most people, but are round numbers). We saw in Chapter 2 that 25 kg of fat could generate 945 MJ on oxidation. So, dividing 945 by about 7.5 gives us 120 days' worth of fat. For people who are initially not overweight, as we might expect, for example, of the Irish hunger strikers, who were prisoners, and especially for males, the starting amount of fat might be half that figure, and we know that Bobby Sands survived for 66 days before succumbing. Gilbert Forbes, a paediatrician at the University of Rochester Medical Center, US, analysed many studies on fasting to develop ways of predicting the loss of fat and muscle: in one of his papers, published in 1970, there is a graph of weight loss of one fasting patient that extends to 132 days (about 19 weeks) (the patient's weight fell from just above 170 kg to about 110 kg). We know that there are many adverse effects of having too much body fat, but one big advantage is clear: the ability to survive starvation for long periods.

Glucose, Insulin, and Fat Mobilisation

Without carbohydrate entering the body, it is essential for the body to economise on glucose utilisation. A key stage of glucose breakdown is the conversion of pyruvic acid (the end-product of the pathway of glycolysis) to acetyl-CoA by the enzyme pyruvate dehydrogenase. Once glucose becomes acetyl-CoA, there is 'no going back': it can no longer be converted back into glucose. In contrast, pyruvic acid can be converted back into glucose (the pathway called gluconeogenesis). So pyruvate dehydrogenase brings about the 'irreversible' breakdown of glucose. It is not surprising, then, that this enzyme is very highly controlled – its activity is influenced by many factors – and it is a key point of regulation in starvation. Its activity is very much suppressed. This means that irreversible loss of glucose from the body is minimised. All tissues that can do so, manage with the pathway of glycolysis, and lactic and pyruvic acids are transferred to the liver to make glucose again – the Cori cycle in operation. This is illustrated in Figure 7.2.

Nevertheless, some glucose continues to be needed for organs that have to oxidise it to gain sufficient energy. The concentration of glucose in the

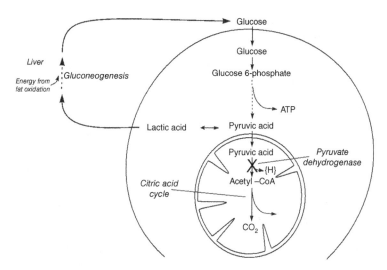

Figure 7.2   Glucose metabolism in starvation. All tissues that can manage just with the pathway of glycolysis do so, and lactic acid is returned to the liver, where it is converted to glucose. This is the Cori cycle, as we saw in Chapter 6. During starvation, the activity of the enzyme pyruvate dehydrogenase is strongly suppressed, so saving glucose from 'irreversible loss' (oxidation to CO_2) in many tissues.

bloodstream drops. In Cahill and Owen's patients, the concentration of glucose in the blood fell from just under 5 mmol/l at the beginning to around 3.7 mmol/l after a few days, and then remained steady. This was accompanied by a fall in the insulin concentration: in the units that they used, falling from 45 (microunits per ml) to 20 after 3 days of fasting, then settling down at about 15.

This fall in insulin concentration has many effects on metabolism. It reduces glucose use by tissues that normally use glucose when insulin is high, muscle in particular. It stimulates the pathway of gluconeogenesis that converts lactic and pyruvic acids back into glucose. This pathway normally operates in the liver: as starvation progresses, it begins to become important also in the kidneys. Falling insulin suppresses the activity of the enzyme pyruvate dehydrogenase responsible for the irreversible loss of glucose, as shown in Figure 7.2.

But perhaps more important are the effects of insulin on our fat stores. Insulin, as we have seen previously, exerts a very powerful restraining influence on fat mobilisation – the release of fatty acids from our fat stores. As the blood insulin concentration falls, fat mobilisation is increased: so the body begins to draw upon its fat stores, as indeed it must to survive without food.

Figure 7.3 shows how glucose, (non-esterified) fatty acid, ketone body and insulin concentrations in the blood changed during starvation in the obese patients studied by Cahill, Owen, and others. (Ketone bodies are explained further below.)

There is a connection here between fat and carbohydrate metabolism. The idea is often expressed that in starvation, protein is broken down to make glucose. That is true – breakdown of some amino acids leads to glucose through the gluconeogenesis pathway, although the sparing of glucose through the recycling mechanism of the Cori cycle is often forgotten. But there is an additional source of material to make new glucose. Each triacyl-glycerol molecule in our fat stores consists of three fatty acid molecules joined to one of glycerol. (Glycerol is a type of alcohol with three carbon atoms.) As fat is mobilised, so fatty acids are released from the fat stores, but so is glycerol, a small, water-soluble compound that is easily transported through the bloodstream to the liver. Glycerol (with three carbon atoms) is a very good substrate for making new glucose in the gluconeogenesis pathway. So some of our fat stores (but not the fatty acids) can be converted to glucose.

Ketone Bodies: Fuel for the Brain

The human brain, as we know, normally uses 100–120 g of glucose per day. How can the brain continue to function when the glycogen reserves have gone, and no new glucose is coming from the intestine? The answer is that the pathway of fat oxidation changes. When fatty acids are oxidised in the liver mitochondria – the pathway of β-oxidation outlined in Chapter 5 – the end-product is once again acetyl-CoA. During normal daily life, most of that acetyl-CoA will be oxidised in the citric acid cycle. But, in liver cells (not in other tissues), some of the acetyl-CoA can be diverted from oxidation into another pathway. Pairs of acetyl-CoA molecules (each with two carbon atoms) can join to make molecules each containing four carbon atoms, called ketone bodies.

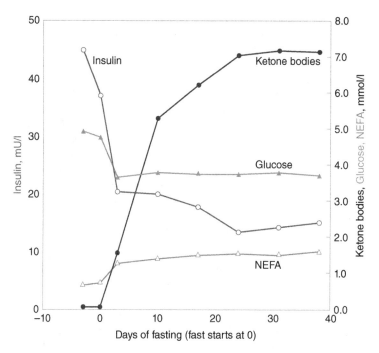

Figure 7.3 Glucose, fatty acid (shown here as 'NEFA', non-esterified fatty acids), ketone body and insulin concentrations in blood plasma during fasting in initially obese patients. Note how the glucose (solid triangles) and insulin (open circles) concentrations fell, while fatty acid (open triangles) and ketone body (solid circles) concentrations increased with time. (Ketone bodies here represent the sum of 3-hydroxybutyrate and acetoacetate concentrations.)

The ketone bodies are always present in our bloodstream but usually at low concentrations, and they don't make much contribution to our metabolism. But their concentration increases when fatty acids are being oxidised in the liver at a high rate. The ketone bodies were at one time thought of as toxic, unwanted waste products. This is because of their association with diabetes, as I shall explain shortly. But now we regard them as key metabolic intermediates, playing a vital role, especially during starvation.

Ketone body production is normally kept in check by insulin. There are two major mechanisms. First, insulin supresses the release of fatty acids from our fat stores (fat mobilisation) as discussed just above. We saw in Chapter 6 how insulin will do this, typically after eating a meal: the body does not need to draw on its fat reserves when nutrients are coming in from the intestine. Secondly, there is a mechanism that we will look at in detail in the next chapter by which a high rate of glucose utilisation (when insulin concentrations are high) prevents fatty acid oxidation. But when the insulin concentration falls, fat mobilisation increases, the supply of fatty acids increases, the pathway for their oxidation increases in activity, and more ketone bodies are formed. Cahill and his colleagues looked at ketone bodies in their fasting patients. A typical pre-starvation level of the ketone bodies (acetoacetate and 3-hydroxybutyrate combined) would be less than 0.2 mmol/l. After 5–6 weeks of starvation, levels of 7–8 mmol/l were found in the patients' blood samples, a 35–40-fold increase, which is quite remarkable for any metabolite in blood (Figure 7.3).

Ketone bodies, produced in the liver, can serve as a fuel for many tissues. Very importantly, they can reach the brain. Normally the brain uses almost exclusively glucose. Fatty acids do not enter the brain to any great extent: they are prevented by the blood–brain barrier, cells lining the brain's blood vessels that prevent toxins getting to the brain. But ketone bodies are not like fatty acids: they are water-soluble (they are not lipids, although they are derived from lipids). So Owen, Cahill, and their colleagues set out to test the idea that ketone bodies might be an important fuel for the brain in starvation.

Nowadays it would be possible to design a radioactive tracer that could be used, with an appropriate imaging technique, to see where ketone bodies are being used in the body. These experimenters used a traditional technique whereby they looked at the blood entering the brain, and the blood leaving the brain, to see what was different: so-called arterio-venous difference measurement. So the patients agreed to have a plastic tube – a catheter – threaded via an artery in the arm, into the aorta near the heart (the main artery of the body, supplying oxygenated blood to all the organs). Another catheter was threaded from a vein in the elbow crease to one of the jugular veins, the large veins in the neck carrying blood away from the brain. All that was done under X-ray control. From these catheters, the experimenters could draw blood samples.

All blood in arteries is the same, as it hasn't yet passed through any tissues, so the experimenters could compare blood from the aorta (assumed to be the same as blood supplying the brain) with blood in a jugular vein leaving the brain. They found that the glucose concentration in the jugular vein was lower than that in the artery: the brain was extracting (using) glucose from the blood. It was also extracting ketone bodies. Assuming that all the glucose and ketone bodies extracted by the brain were oxidised, then glucose was supplying one third of the brain's energy requirement, and the ketone bodies two thirds.

This quite remarkable piece of experimentation has shown clearly a key feature of the metabolic adaptation that allows humans to starve for long periods. Our fat stores are our largest energy reserve. But the brain cannot use fatty acids as a fuel. Instead, fatty acids are converted in the liver to ketone bodies and then the brain can use them, and this spares the body's glucose reserves.

Starvation and Diabetes Contrasted

You have probably read about ketone bodies before. When ketone body concentrations in blood are high, that state is referred to loosely as ketosis. As I have said, at one time doctors regarded ketone bodies as toxic waste products. Now dieters praise them and consider a state of ketosis to be something like nirvana. For sure, elevated ketone body concentrations show that the body is oxidising its fat stores. But if it weren't doing that, it would be oxidising something else. There is anecdotal evidence that a high ketone body concentration in blood reduces appetite. I don't think that's ever been formally tested, but it would make sense of the fact that people who starve – or who starve themselves of carbohydrate, to induce ketosis – claim not to have a great feeling of hunger, at least once the metabolic situation has adapted. (The Minnesota volunteers would be surprised to hear of this: it might be because they were only semi-starved that they did not experience this relief from intense hunger.)

The reason for the previous toxic reputation of ketone bodies is their association with poorly treated type 1 diabetes, which is caused by a lack of insulin (because of an auto-immune process that destroys the β-cells of the Islets of Langerhans that secrete insulin). I described earlier how a low insulin concentration will lead to increased fatty acid release from fat stores, and increased ketone body formation. When there is essentially no insulin, these processes are greatly increased. If someone with type 1 diabetes does not, for whatever reason, receive adequate insulin treatment, then within a very few days ketone body concentrations will increase to the sort of levels we saw in long-term starvation – say around 8 mmol/l, although they can be considerably more. This medical situation is called diabetic ketoacidosis. It is a life-threatening situation. Patients will die unless given insulin. A very typical story would be that a patient becomes ill, for instance with an infection, doesn't feel well, and thinks perhaps it would be wise not to inject insulin today. But actually the body probably needs more insulin than usual in that situation. Within 24 hours the patient may be feeling seriously poorly and perhaps, with luck, within 36–48 hours is admitted to hospital – and a good doctor will then quickly see what is wrong and institute the necessary treatment. If the patient doesn't reach hospital, or arrives too late, this is still a fatal situation. When blood ketone body concentrations are very high, an additional product is acetone (a ketone body with three carbon atoms, formed spontaneously by loss of carbon dioxide). Acetone is present in the breath, with a characteristic smell (like nail-varnish remover). It used to be said that a good physician could walk onto the ward, smell the acetone in the air and demand 'Show me the case of diabetic ketoacidosis.'

But here is my metabolic point, and this is a puzzle I have posed for biochemistry students many times. How come a ketone body concentration of 7 or 8 mmol/l is life-threatening to someone with diabetes – but allows a fasting patient to survive? What's the difference? We'll see the answer when we have looked, in the next section, at amino acid metabolism.

Protein and Amino Acid Metabolism in Fasting

We have seen that a slowing down of amino acid breakdown is one of the key adaptations to starvation, sparing the body's proteins. The exact mechanisms that bring this about are unclear. Normally a falling insulin concentration would be expected to increase protein breakdown, and hence amino acid oxidation, so something is working against this. The falling concentration of the thyroid hormone T_3 may be involved: normally a high concentration of T_3 would tend to increase muscle protein breakdown. Of the other specific mechanisms that have been proposed, one is of interest here: a high concentration of ketone bodies is a signal to muscle to spare its protein stores. There is some, albeit limited, experimental evidence for this.

There are clear changes in the pattern of amino acid metabolism in starvation. One marked effect is that the kidneys become very involved, especially with utilisation of the amino acid glutamine. Glutamine is the amino acid present at the highest concentration in blood. It is, like alanine, an amino acid released in relatively large amounts from muscle. An enzyme called glutaminase is responsible for removing one of the two nitrogen-containing groups from glutamine. We have two versions of the enzyme glutaminase, coded for by different, but related, genes. One form is important in the liver, feeding nitrogen from amino acids into the synthesis of urea, for excretion in the urine. The kidney form, on the other hand, splits a nitrogen-containing group (an amide group) from glutamine, forming ammonia (NH_3) and leaving the amino acid glutamic acid. Ammonia may then be excreted in the urine. In this case, it takes with it a hydrogen ion (H^+) to form the ammonium ion NH_4^+. The gene for this kidney form of glutaminase is activated when the blood becomes acid: more copies of the protein (the enzyme) are made, and this takes several days to become maximal. Acids are characterised by a hydrogen atom that can come off as an ion, H^+. The body needs to control the acidity of the blood – measured on the scale called pH. One way it can do this is by excreting excess hydrogen ions, H^+, from the kidney as ammonium, NH_4^+. (The glutamic acid that results from splitting glutamine in the kidney can then be used to make new glucose – this is one reason the kidneys in starvation begin to contribute to new glucose production, along with the liver.)

Now to come back to the puzzle about why diabetic ketoacidosis is so much more dangerous than the ketosis of starvation. Both are characterised by high concentrations of the ketone bodies 3-hydroxybutyric acid and acetoacetic acid, and also the non-esterified fatty acids from adipose tissue. These substances are all acids. If their concentration rises rapidly, as it does in diabetes, then the body has not had time to up-regulate its capacity to get rid of the excess acid. The increased acidity of the blood becomes very dangerous – hence the term diabetic keto*acidosis*. In starvation, on the other hand, things happen much more slowly. Ketone body concentrations rise over a period of 2–3 weeks. Kidney glutaminase is up-regulated, and the acidity is kept under control.

Slow and Fast Metabolism

Now we have seen an example of 'slow metabolism' – whole-body energy expenditure is reduced in starvation so as to prolong the time that the body can keep going. Next we will look at a situation in which metabolism is clearly speeded up – physical activity.

Exercise and Physical Activity

Experts in the field would distinguish between the terms 'physical activity' and 'exercise'. Both imply that the body is exerting a force to do external work. Dylan Thompson, Professor of Human Physiology at the University of Bath, has written: 'Physical activity is defined as any movement (or force) exerted by skeletal muscle that leads to an increase in energy expenditure above rest. Exercise is usually described as a subcomponent of physical activity that is planned and/or structured'.

We are all advised to maintain physical activity for the sake of our health. In the UK, Government guidelines are that adults should perform at least 30 minutes of moderate intensity activity on at least 5 days a week. Moderate intensity is defined as a three-fold increase in metabolic rate above rest. But Dylan Thompson has made some very interesting observations that bear on just how this is brought about. Some people lead active lifestyles without necessarily engaging in bouts of structured exercise. Others engage in structured exercise but, other than that, spend long periods sedentary. We really don't know the implications of those different patterns for health.

There are two distinct ways of expressing the intensity of physical activity. One is to measure the rate of doing external work. A stationary exercise cycle may be calibrated in watts (W), for instance, showing how much work is being done. But we can also look at the energy expenditure of the person doing the work, measured through oxygen consumption and carbon dioxide production. These two ways of measuring work will not be the same – like any mechanical device, the human body is not 100% efficient in translating its fuel use into external work. A very typical figure would be that the external work done is about one quarter of the total energy expenditure – a mechanical efficiency of around 25%, the rest being liberated directly as heat.

One convenient way of expressing the energy cost of various activities is by expressing the person's energy expenditure in relation to his or her energy

Activity	Energy expenditure (metabolic rate), MET
Resting (not asleep)	1.0
Sleeping	0.9
Light housework (e.g. sweeping the floor)	2.5
Walking steadily (3 miles/hour or 5 kilometres/hour)	3.5
Heavy housework (e.g. washing car, mopping the floor)	4.5
Dancing	3–7
Swimming	6–11
Strenuous hill-walking (averaged over a whole walk including rests)	9
Jogging	10–12
Playing squash	12
Marathon running	18

One MET is defined as the normal resting metabolic rate (i.e. whole-body energy expenditure at rest). It is about 4.8 kJ/min for a man of average size, and 3.8 kJ/min for a woman of average size. Note that 4.8 kJ/min is 4 800/60 J/sec, = 80 W (about the heat output of an incandescent light bulb). Remember that the figures given are for total energy expenditure by the body; the amount of *external work* done will be about one quarter of this (since the body as a machine has an efficiency of about 25%).

The figures in this table are, of course, approximations only.

Collated from various sources; reproduced from Frayn, K. N. & Evans, R. D. (2019). *Human Metabolism: A Regulatory Perspective*, 4th edn. Oxford: Wiley Blackwell.

Table 7.1   Energy expenditure during various activities

expenditure at rest (the so-called resting metabolic rate). Table 7.1 shows the energy costs measured in this way of various forms of physical activity.

Muscles

Physical activity means using muscles to do work. There are different sorts of muscle. The muscles that we use for work are called skeletal muscles, because they attach to the skeleton to move our bones. There are also muscles lining our blood vessels and intestines, over which we have no direct control: these are called smooth muscles because of their appearance under the microscope. And there is the muscle of the heart – the heart is essentially a muscular organ, pumping blood through the lungs to acquire oxygen and give up carbon dioxide, and then around the rest of the body. Heart muscle is called cardiac muscle: the organ itself is called the myocardium (*myo* meaning to do with muscle). Here we shall mainly be looking at skeletal muscles, the muscles over which we have conscious control, although many features of myocardial metabolism are similar.

If you look at a cross-section of a skeletal muscle under the microscope, you see that it is made up of individual fibres. These fibres are muscle cells. (They are complex cells made from the fusion of precursor cells, and each has more than one nucleus.) You can see some in Figure 7.4.

Each of these fibres is packed with proteins in the form of long strands called fibrils. Muscle is, indeed, composed largely of protein, nearly one quarter of its weight (most of the rest is water). Hence, as I have mentioned before, muscle is by far the largest reservoir of protein in the human body. Two of these proteins, called actin and myosin, make up the bulk, and they form strands that run between each other. Contraction of a muscle consists of the filaments of these two proteins, actin and myosin, moving relative to each other. That process requires energy since it will generate a force, and each step of the filaments over each other is accompanied by the use of one molecule of ATP (the energy-carrying molecule that we discussed in detail in Chapter 5). It is initiated by an increase in the local concentration of calcium, in the form of charged atoms (ions, written as Ca^{2+}).

When we decide to move a muscle, a signal is sent from the brain along the appropriate motor neuron, and reaches the muscle. That nerve releases a transmitter substance called acetylcholine, which binds to receptors on the muscle cell, triggering a release of Ca^{2+} ions in the vicinity of the contractile proteins. The protein filaments then move relative to one another, accompanied by use of ATP. (When the ATP is used, it becomes ADP – adenosine diphosphate – and normally goes back to the mitochondria, that are plentiful in skeletal muscle, to be made back into ATP.) Nerve agents, incidentally, interfere with signalling by acetylcholine, thus paralysing the muscles.

Metabolic changes in muscle are amongst the most dramatic of any situation we are likely to encounter, unless we meet with a sudden accident. The flow of material through the pathway of glucose breakdown (glycolysis) may

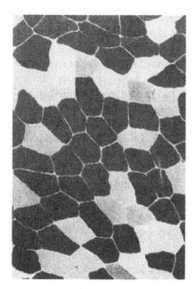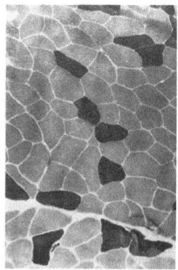

Figure 7.4 Muscle fibres.
Cross-sections through human leg muscles. The polygon shapes are individual muscles cells, also called muscle fibres. Here they are stained to show different types of muscle fibre, as explained in the text. The dark-stained fibres are the type 2 (fast-twitch) fibres, the lighter ones the type 1 (slow-twitch) fibres. These samples are taken from two athletes: on the left, a high jumper, and on the right, a marathon runner. The marathon runner compared with the high jumper has a much greater proportion of slow-twitch fibres. This is essentially something they inherit – training cannot change this much. So the person whose muscle is shown on the right was born to be a long-distance runner and would not be good at an explosive sport such as high jump. Typical muscle fibres are 20–100 μm across (where 100 μm is 0.1 mm).

increase something like 1 000-fold within a second or two. When muscle contraction stops, flow through glycolysis can switch back to baseline within a similar timeframe. Such changes illustrate the power of metabolic regulation.

Fast-twitch Muscles

Muscles can generate force without any metabolic input from the rest of the body, which makes for very rapid contraction. Everything that is needed is present within the muscle fibre (the cell). There are some muscle fibres that are specialised to do this. When we looked at muscle structure in Figure 7.4, we saw the different sorts of fibre (they can be stained to appear light and dark under the microscope, as in the figure). The muscle fibres that are specialised to conduct this rapid contraction do not need to use oxygen, so they do not have many mitochondria, and they mostly lack the red protein called myoglobin (related to haemoglobin) that helps conduct oxygen into the cells. They appear pale, and are known generally as white muscle fibres. Technically these are often called type 2 muscle fibres, or fast-twitch muscle fibres, since they can contract so quickly. In many animals, whole muscles are made mainly of one type of muscle fibre: hence if you eat a chicken, you can choose 'light' or 'dark' meat (mainly white or red muscle). In rodents, you can see with the naked eye that some of the muscles are very pale, others much redder. In humans, in contrast, most muscles have a mixture of fibres, although the proportions will differ between individuals, as shown in Figure 7.4.

These white, or type 2, muscle fibres have two means by which they can generate energy quickly. The first is this. In addition to ATP, these fibres contain another compound with a 'high-energy' phosphate group. This is creatine phosphate (or phosphocreatine). Creatine is, chemically, an amino acid, although it has a rather different structure from those amino acids that are incorporated into proteins. Creatine phosphate is made from creatine by an enzyme called creatine kinase (a kinase being an enzyme that adds a phosphate group from ATP). That reaction can also run in the other direction:

Creatine + ATP ↔ Creatine phosphate + ADP

White muscle fibres contain about three to four times as much creatine phosphate as ATP. So this is a 'buffer' for the ATP store. As soon as ATP is used in muscle contraction, the ADP is rephosphorylated (converted back to ATP) using the high-energy phosphate group of creatine phosphate:

Creatine phosphate + ADP → Creatine + ATP

This extends the time that the muscle can keep contracting before these high-energy stores are depleted, when they must be topped up from glycogen breakdown and glycolysis. When the muscle rests again, ATP can be made from other sources, and the creatine phosphate store can be rebuilt – the reaction runs in the opposite direction. In experimental studies in which volunteers use their legs to do heavy work against a resistance while an experimenter from time to time plunges in a needle to take a sample of muscle, the concentration of ATP will stay fairly constant for perhaps 20 seconds, while the concentration of creatine phosphate decreases steadily to almost zero. Our cells can make creatine from the amino acid arginine. But taking creatine as a dietary supplement will increase the muscle store, with benefits for athletes in sprint-type events: it does not help endurance athletes, whose muscles are deriving energy in different ways.

As the creatine phosphate store is depleted, another mechanism is coming into play. Muscles, as we have seen, contain their own store of glycogen. The release of calcium ions that triggers muscle contraction also activates the enzyme that breaks down glycogen (glycogen phosphorylase). This liberates glucose 6-phosphate, that can enter the pathway of glycolysis. We saw in Chapter 5 that breakdown of glucose by the pathway of glycolysis makes some ATP: the process called substrate-level phosphorylation, not involving the mitochondria. This can all happen extremely rapidly upon activation of the muscles through the nerves. It does not involve hormones, and it does not require anything to be brought to the muscle through the bloodstream: oxygen is not needed, and carbon dioxide is not produced, because the pyruvic acid, which is the end-product of glycolysis, may not be further oxidised in this scenario: in fact, it will be converted to lactic acid, which will begin to build up.

This form of muscle contraction is called anaerobic, because it does not need oxygen. It is the type of muscle contraction used for very rapid, strenuous bursts of exercise such as short sprints (e.g. 100 metres) and for explosive events like jumping. But it cannot keep us going for long. The creatine phosphate store is soon depleted, and as lactic acid and other metabolites accumulate in the muscle, this begins to put a brake on further glycolysis. (This used to be ascribed to increasing acidity in the muscles, but is now thought to be due more to accumulation of phosphate, P_i, from use of creatine phosphate.)

Slow-twitch Muscles

In order to keep muscles contracting for longer periods, we need to bring in additional fuels, and oxygen, through the bloodstream. As the muscles begin full oxidation of their nutrients, lactic acid accumulation decreases (because the pyruvic acid from glycolysis can be oxidised in the mitochondria, through the citric acid cycle). What is more, you will remember from Chapter 5 that complete oxidation of glucose via this route generates far more ATP than the substrate-level phosphorylation that happens in glycolysis.

This oxidative metabolism is a property of distinct muscle fibres, that appear darker because of the presence of many mitochondria, and the protein myoglobin that helps transfer the oxygen through the cell. They are called red muscle fibres, or type 1, or slow-twitch. These muscle fibres can keep contracting for very long periods. The oxygen and the fuel they need come through the bloodstream – e.g. glucose from the glycogen store in the liver, fatty acids from the fat stores – and because of the role of the bloodstream, waste products (carbon dioxide and lactic acid) can be removed as they are formed. But oxidative metabolism of fuels is necessarily a slower process than the rapid anaerobic metabolism we considered earlier: oxygen and fuels must diffuse from the capillaries of the circulation to where they are needed; waste products must diffuse back out. So the role of this type of muscle fibre, and its oxidative metabolism, is to enable exercise to be conducted for much longer periods, although not at the same intensity: the marathon runner cannot run as fast as the sprinter, but can keep going for much longer.

You may have come across the terms 'anaerobic exercise' and 'aerobic exercise': these are the metabolic processes that underlie these different types of exercise.

Communications during Exercise

Clearly the nervous system is intimately involved in the process of muscle contraction: signals through motor neurons stimulate the muscles to contract. Hormones are also involved. Adrenaline is released from the adrenal medulla and helps with the breakdown of glycogen even in anaerobic exercise (through the mechanism shown in Figure 4.2). As exercise continues, then adrenaline and the sympathetic nervous system play bigger roles. They stimulate the heart to pump harder, so delivering more blood to the muscles. Blood flow through the muscles increases concomitantly. It was at one time thought that the sympathetic nervous system was responsible for that, but now it seems more likely that it is caused by compounds released locally from the contracting muscles. Adrenaline, and probably the sympathetic nerves, also lead to the activation of fuel mobilisation: glycogen breakdown in the liver, so releasing glucose for the muscles, and fat mobilisation in the adipose depots (fat stores), so delivering fatty acids. In prolonged exercise (an hour or more) it is likely that other hormones begin to play a role in driving fat mobilisation, including cortisol and growth hormone.

Fuels Used during Exercise

During short bursts of intense exercise, once creatine phosphate has been depleted, the fuel used is mainly glycogen stored within the muscle fibres. This will be rebuilt when exercise stops, when carbohydrate is available (e.g. after eating, so providing glucose and a rise in insulin concentration).

Much of our understanding of the role of muscle glycogen during exercise stems from the work of two individuals. Eric Hultman was a Swedish physiologist, who, to help his research, had developed a very sensitive method for measuring small amounts of glycogen. He got together with Jonas Bergström, a Swedish kidney doctor, who had developed a hollow needle that could be used to take small samples from someone's muscle. Between them, they published many scientific papers on muscle glycogen and exercise. Many of the early studies of Eric Hultman and Jonas Bergström were based on observations and experiments in just two people, and it should not have taken me by surprise, when I got to know their work, to find in one of their papers that the data from these two subjects were labelled 'EH' and 'JB'. Like many pioneering experimenters, they had found it easiest to use themselves as guinea pigs.

So, as we have seen, muscle glycogen is used during muscle contractions. To what extent is the breakdown of glycogen due to hormones, and to what extent is it due to factors operating within the exercising muscle? To answer this, Hultman and Bergström constructed an exercise cycle with just one pedal: so, one leg of the experimental volunteer would exercise, whilst the other was at rest. If a hormone (such as adrenaline) were the trigger for glycogen breakdown, then both legs should be affected equally. But – by taking samples from the muscles of both legs at intervals – they found that the resting leg's glycogen content did not change, whilst that in the exercising leg went down to almost zero (Figure 7.5). So clearly factors within the muscle are the more important, as I described earlier – although we would believe now that adrenaline, acting on in concert with the contraction process, probably

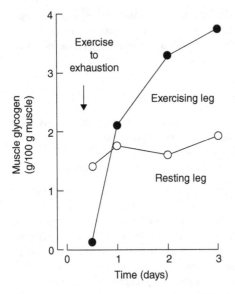

Figure 7.5 Glycogen concentrations in leg muscle after one-legged exercise (bicycling on a specially adapted bicycle), in the exercised leg (solid points) and the non-exercised leg (open points). Average of two subjects.

does have a role. But this experiment had a remarkable spin-off. They continued to take muscle samples daily for 3 days after the exercise, and found that glycogen in the leg that had exercised jumped back much beyond its starting level – a phenomenon they called 'supercompensation'.

Hultman and Bergström's studies illustrated the important role of muscle glycogen during exercise. They showed very clearly that exhaustion – when an experimental volunteer in the exercise laboratory could just not go on any longer – was the point of depletion of the muscle glycogen store. Further, they showed that muscle glycogen stores could be manipulated by diet – a carbohydrate-rich diet would raise muscle glycogen levels compared with a fat-rich (and hence carbohydrate-poor) diet, and this enabled subjects to exercise for longer before exhaustion. Those observations led to the now-universal practice of 'glycogen loading' by endurance athletes before an event. In the original form of glycogen loading, the athlete would exercise to exhaustion a few days before the event, then eat a carbohydrate-rich diet, so leading to supercompensation and high glycogen levels before the start of the event. Now the exercise to exhaustion is not thought to be so important, but pre-event carbohydrate loading is still the norm

But there is a paradox here. Glycogen stores are limited: fat stores are virtually unlimited. Why should endurance exercise rely on the glycogen stores? A consensus answer would be along these lines. Certainly muscles can generate energy for contraction by oxidising fatty acids. But it seems that this can never be as fast a route of ATP generation as glucose oxidation. There are many reasons for that: fatty acids need to be brought to the muscles from adipose tissue, and, since they are not directly water-soluble, they need to be carried on the protein albumin, and so perhaps can't get out of the adipose tissue fast enough; within the muscles, diffusion of fatty acids to the site of oxidation may be slower than that of water-soluble glucose. And there may also be a metabolic interaction, that we shall look at in the next chapter, that reduces fatty acid oxidation when glucose is being used at a high rate. Hence, elite marathon runners rely on starting a race with sufficient glycogen stores to see them through to the end. If glycogen stores run out, then the athlete experiences the phenomenon known as 'hitting the wall': fat oxidation takes over, but at a slower pace, and the athlete has to slow down.

But fat oxidation can indeed be a good fuel source for muscles: just not at the same rate as carbohydrates. During fairly low intensity exercise, fat is the main fuel for muscle contraction. Also, in prolonged exercise – running more than the marathon distance – fat is, of necessity, the main fuel. Elite ultra-marathoners, running distances of 50 km or more, cannot run as fast as elite marathoners – but they can keep going for a lot longer by using their fat stores.

Fat is especially important for exercise at relatively low intensities. This was beautifully illustrated in a study performed by John Wahren and colleagues, in Stockholm and at Yale University in the US. The experimenters inserted a fine plastic catheter into a femoral artery (the artery supplying blood to the leg). They put a similar catheter into a femoral vein, the large vein that carries the blood away from the leg. By drawing blood samples from the catheters in the femoral artery and vein, the experimenters could see what metabolites were being used by the muscles in the leg. (This is the same principle as used by

Oliver Owen, George Cahill, and others to study fuels used by the brain in starvation.) For instance, the glucose concentration was less in the vein than the artery, because the muscles were extracting glucose from the blood. They could also measure uptake of oxygen in the leg (by measuring the concentration of oxygen in the blood in the artery and vein), and uptake of fatty acids, although that required also use of an isotope tracer (because in the leg there are both adipose tissues, releasing fatty acids, and muscles, using them). The six volunteers then exercised on a stationary bicycle for 4 hours. The intensity of exercise was calculated as '30% of maximal oxygen uptake', which is not very strenuous, but no doubt felt so as the hours went on. The results are shown in Figure 7.6.

Even early on, fatty acids made a greater contribution to leg exercise than glucose, and this increased steadily as exercise progressed. These fatty acids were supplied, of course, by increased delivery from the fat stores (mostly outside the leg).

People who exercise early in the morning, before their breakfast, will also be largely using fat along with glycogen that was stored in their muscles. From studies such as this one, the idea has arisen of so-called fat-burning exercise, implying that certain types and intensities of exercise, and certain times of day for exercise, will preferentially use fat as a fuel (which is undoubtedly true), and therefore will be more beneficial in terms of losing weight. If you are a believer in this idea, then I am sorry to say that I am not, and I will explain my reasons more in the next chapter when we consider relationships between carbohydrate and fat metabolism. But to summarise here, my own belief – based upon experimental work both from my own research group and others – is that exercise uses energy, and in the long term it doesn't matter if the immediate fuel is carbohydrate or fat – they both contribute to a loss of fuel from the body's fuel stores. You might want to argue that types of exercise that use predominantly glycogen [short, high-intensity exercise, for instance] do not therefore impinge upon the body's fat stores. But that is to fundamentally misunderstand just how closely energy, fat, and carbohydrate metabolism are inter-related. We will explore this more in the next chapter.

To finish this section, we'll just ask the question: how much ATP is used during a typical marathon run? To answer it, you need to know various things, including the typical energy cost of running a marathon, which is around

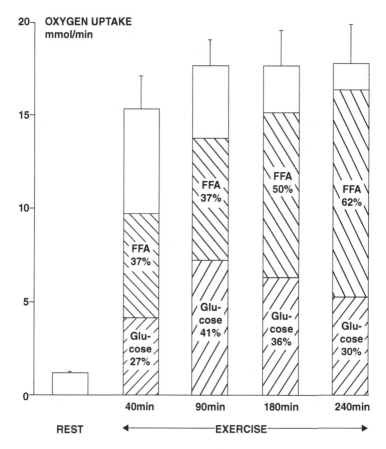

Figure 7.6   Metabolic fuels used by exercising legs.

The volunteers, Stockholm firemen, cycled for 4 hours at low-to-moderate intensity. Blood samples were drawn from the artery supplying the leg and the vein draining it to see what was being used. The total height of each bar is the oxygen consumed by the leg. You can see how it increases about 10-fold from rest to exercise. The contributions of fatty acids (shown as 'FFA', free fatty acids) and glucose are expressed as their contribution to leg oxygen consumption. The remainder, shown as a white bar, is assumed to be mainly from muscle glycogen with perhaps some contribution from fat stored in the muscles. Note how the contribution of fatty acids (FFA) increases with time, but is always greater than that of glucose at this intensity of exercise.

10–12.5 MJ (say 2 500–3 000 kcal). The answer, depending on exactly how the calculation is done, turns out to be about 65 kg of ATP – similar to the body weight of many marathon runners! Clearly the athlete does not start out with 65 kg of ATP in his or her muscles. There is a very small amount – but it is continually used (making ADP) and resynthesised (from ADP) during the exercise, using the energy liberated by oxidation of carbohydrate and fat.

Fight or Flight

The term 'fight or flight response' is often bandied around. Since it has some connections with exercise, we will look at it here. The term was coined by the American physiologist and physician Walter Cannon in the 1920s, but Cannon had begun his research in this area much earlier, and in 1915 had published the book *Bodily Changes in Pain, Hunger, Fear and Rage*. He worked in field hospitals during the First World War studying 'wound shock', so he had plenty of direct knowledge of the body's responses to trauma. Cannon recognised that the response to sudden stress was to increase the activity of the sympathetic nervous system, and that this was accompanied by increased liberation of the hormone adrenaline (adrenin, as he called it then, now called epinephrine in the US). The effect of these changes is to mobilise the body's fuel stores, increase the heart rate, and open up some blood vessels: just the preparation needed if the person affected is about to engage in physical combat, or indeed flee the scene.

Just as occurs during exercise, fuel mobilisation in the fight or flight response consists of glycogen breakdown – liberating glucose, ready for use by the muscles – and fat mobilisation, liberating fatty acids. A case has been made that these changes account for the adverse health effects of stress. In the fight or flight situation, these fuels will be used for muscular work. If the stress is there without the physical activity, they will accumulate in the bloodstream. Very high levels of these non-esterified fatty acids have been measured, for instance, in people at public speaking events, and in racing drivers just before a race. Elevated concentrations of the non-esterified fatty acids can have immediate adverse effects, including disturbing the heart rhythm and promoting blood clotting. The late British biochemist Eric Newsholme, in his book *Biochemistry for the Medical Sciences* (written with Tony Leech), suggested that this may be a factor in heart attacks sometimes suffered by airline pilots, including the pilot of a British European Airways flight that crashed after take-off from London Heathrow in 1972: it was known that this pilot was involved in a heated argument shortly before take-off.

Carbohydrates and Fats as Fuels

So we have seen how both carbohydrates and fats have roles in providing fuel for muscular work. One or the other will predominate according to the circumstances. But that does not mean that they operate independently of one another. Indeed, the connections between carbohydrate and fat metabolism are particularly intimate. Since this has been the cause of much confusion, it will be the subject of our next chapter.

8 Metabolic Interactions between Nutrients

Carbohydrate, Fat, and Amino Acid Metabolism Are Necessarily Inter-connected

Over 10 years, those of us eating diets typical of Western societies will eat around 1 tonne (1 000 kg) of carbohydrate, and 250–300 kg each of protein and fat. Yet, for many of us, our bodies will change little (maybe a few kg extra or less, but that's a tiny percentage of what we take in). It just seems unarguable that the body must have ways of adjusting the use (oxidation) of each nutrient in relation to our energy needs, and in relation to other nutrients. And yet many people seem not to believe this. In this chapter we will look at how these nutrients interact metabolically, and (briefly) at some ramifications for what we eat.

Energy Is the Primary Determinant: Fuel Use Adjusts according to Availability

We can see how this may happen from the results of a very simple experiment conducted by Helen Whitley, a student working in my laboratory in Oxford (in collaboration with colleagues at the Universities of Manchester and Liverpool John Moores).

Helen recruited a group of volunteers, who came to the laboratory on three occasions, each time having fasted overnight. In the laboratory, they were given one of three different meals, with very different proportions of carbohydrate and fat – protein was kept constant, as was the energy content. To quote from the paper we published on the results, and to give an idea of how such experiments are designed, 'The constituents for meals 1, 2 and 3 were chosen to typify a breakfast cereal, comprising oats, coconut, almonds, raisins, honey, sunflower oil, banana, double cream and milk, and were selected to resemble each other both in appearance and palatability'. Helen worked all that out on a spreadsheet, juggling the proportions of the ingredients to obtain the amounts of carbohydrate and fat she required. She made measurements before the breakfast. Then, during the next 5 hours, she drew regular blood samples, and connected the volunteers to an indirect calorimetry apparatus (to measure oxygen consumption and carbon dioxide production). This enabled her to measure how much energy was being expended, and also, by examination of the ratio of oxygen consumption to carbon dioxide production, the contributions of carbohydrate and fat oxidation to energy expenditure. (Box 8.1 below explains how this works.) The results are shown in Figure 8.1.

The numbers below the graph show the amount of carbohydrate and fat in each meal, so they ranged from a high-carbohydrate/low fat meal (Meal 1) to a high-fat/low carbohydrate meal (Meal 3). The bars show 'balance': that is, the amount stored in the body, calculated as the amount consumed minus the amount expended or oxidised over 5 hours. The bars represent, in order, carbohydrate (shaded), fat (white), and energy (black). The volunteers all

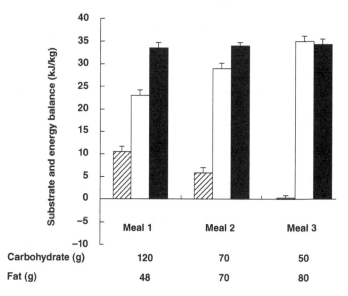

Figure 8.1 Carbohydrate and fat balance after meals of different composition
The graph is explained in the text.

ended up with an excess of energy, which was almost exactly equal after each of the meals (black bars). But this energy excess was made up from carbohydrate and fat in varying proportions according to the content of the meal: there was, as we put it in the paper, 'an inverse relationship between carbohydrate and fat balance following these meals, with carbohydrate balance decreasing as carbohydrate intake decreased, and fat balance increasing as fat intake increased'.

In short, despite different amounts of carbohydrate and fat taken in for breakfast, the same amount of energy was expended, but made up of differing proportions of carbohydrate and fat. Clearly, metabolic mechanisms within the body adjusted carbohydrate and fat oxidation according to their availability, whilst energy expenditure was constant.

The fact that carbohydrate and fat interact metabolically has been known for many years – perhaps, we might say, since the 1960s when the regulation of fat mobilisation became clear; but now we understand a host of mechanisms that operate to manage their relationship. Another way of looking at this is to recognise that, as we saw in Chapter 5, both carbohydrate and fat, along with amino acids and other nutrients such as alcohol, feed into a common cellular pool of acetyl-CoA, which then feeds into the citric acid cycle. The citric acid cycle has a fixed capacity – partly fixed by the rate at which ATP is used, hence releasing ADP to make new ATP. It is inevitable that if one nutrient is present in excess, the breakdown of another must be modulated appropriately.

Box 8.1 The principles of human calorimetry.

Calorimetry means measurement of heat. It is possible to measure the output of heat from the human body. (Heat output, from a resting person, is effectively their energy expenditure.) This involves constructing a well-insulated box or chamber in which a person can spend some time. In the walls of the chamber, or calorimeter, are electrical thermocouples to measure temperature, or alternatively pipes through which water is passed, so that the increase in temperature of the water may be measured. These procedures are extremely demanding experimentally, and not often employed.

An alternative is to calculate heat production, or energy expenditure, by measuring how much oxygen is being used. This was the technique used by Lavoisier (Figure 1.1). This can be done by enclosing the person in a chamber, or by collecting the expired air through a mask or a hood over the subject's head and analysing the composition of the incoming and outgoing air. The amount of heat associated with each litre of oxygen used is known from other experimental work. Because this is an indirect measure of heat output, it is known as indirect calorimetry.

The amount of heat associated with each litre of oxygen depends slightly upon which metabolic fuels are being used. A refinement is to measure, in addition, the production of carbon dioxide. Measurement of oxygen consumption and carbon dioxide production combined gives an accurate measure of energy expenditure. Figure 8.2 shows a modern indirect calorimetry apparatus.

But the technique of indirect calorimetry has a further advantage: it gives information on the metabolic fuels being used.

If we write the equation for oxidation of glucose, it is:

$$C_6H_{12}O_6 + 6O_2 \rightarrow 6CO_2 + 6H_2O$$

Gases occupy volumes that depend on the number of molecules present. In this case, the volume of carbon dioxide (CO_2) produced will be the same as the volume of oxygen (O_2) consumed, since equal numbers of molecules are involved. The ratio of these volumes is called the respiratory quotient (usually abbreviated to RQ). In this case the RQ is 1.0.

But if we write a similar equation for oxidation of fat, it is different. This equation looks messy because it depends whether we are talking about fatty acids or triacylglycerols, and also which particular fatty acids are being oxidised. But typically, for a triacylglycerol:

$$C_{55}H_{104}O_6 + 78O_2 \rightarrow 55CO_2 + 52H_2O$$

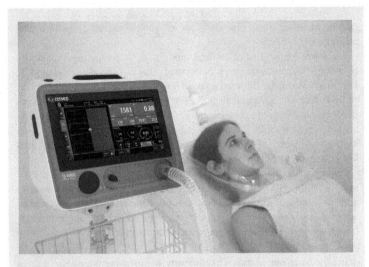

Figure 8.2 Measurement of oxygen consumption and carbon dioxide production using a portable indirect calorimeter.

In this case, the RQ is 55/78, or 0.71. So, if we measure the RQ carefully, we can work out the proportions of fat and carbohydrate being used.

In a further refinement, we can allow for the oxidation of amino acids. This can be done by measuring the amount of nitrogen (mainly in urea) excreted in the urine, since oxidation of amino acids must lead to excretion of their nitrogen content.

It is also possible to attribute a Respiratory Quotient, RQ, to other metabolic processes. The process of lipogenesis, synthesis of fat from glucose, has an RQ greater than 1.0. If ever the RQ measured for the whole body (sometimes called the Respiratory Exchange Ratio, RER) exceeds 1.0, we know that fat is being made *in a net sense* from glucose.

Glucose Can Make Fat, but Fat Can't Make Glucose

A very fundamental way in which glucose and fat interact is this: spare glucose can be made into fat, whereas the opposite is not true. The pathway of making new fatty acids is called lipogenesis – usually, to make clear that it means making new fatty acids from other substances, it is qualified as *de novo* lipogenesis. The pathway has long been understood. Acetyl-CoA that may come from glucose, amino acids, or alcohol is the starting point. Further acetyl-CoA units (with two carbon atoms) are added sequentially to create the fatty acid palmitic acid, with 16 carbon atoms and no unsaturation – it is a saturated fatty acid. In the body, though, as we saw earlier, much of the palmitic acid will feed through into the pathway called desaturation, which will convert it to an unsaturated fatty acid. Desaturation is also linked to the pathway called elongation, in which further acetyl-CoA units can be added. Thus, for instance, oleic acid (18 carbons, mono-unsaturated) can be made by these pathways operating sequentially.

This pathway is slightly more complicated than I have made it sound. Acetyl-CoA from glucose, fatty acid, or amino acid breakdown is formed within mitochondria, whereas the pathway of lipogenesis takes place in the cytoplasm of the cell – outside the mitochondria. A series of reactions has the net effect of transferring acetyl-CoA from inside the mitochondrion to the cytoplasm. And in the pathway of lipogenesis, it's not acetyl-CoA directly that adds two-carbon units. The acetyl-CoA is changed, by addition of carbon dioxide (which is present in solution in the cell), into a compound called malonyl-CoA. Malonyl-CoA therefore has three carbon atoms (plus the coenzyme-A). But as it is joined to the growing fatty acid chain, one is lost again (converted back to carbon dioxide), so two carbons are added. Why did I mention this complication? Because it's fundamental to control of the pathway, as we shall see. The enzyme that converts acetyl-CoA and carbon dioxide to malonyl-CoA is called acetyl-CoA carboxylase.

There are six different reactions to make malonyl-CoA into fatty acids. In bacteria, this is done by six different enzymes. But in mammals, these functions have fused into one complex enzyme, called fatty acid synthase, produced from one gene, called (in humans) *FASN*. Therefore, just two enzymes are involved in making fatty acids from acetyl-CoA: acetyl-CoA carboxylase and fatty acid synthase. You can see this schematically in Figure 3.4.

This pathway, the conversion of glucose to fat via acetyl-CoA, is stimulated by insulin. That stimulation occurs at many steps. In some tissues, for instance adipose tissue (fat storage tissue), glucose entry into the cells is stimulated by insulin. Glycolysis is also stimulated by insulin, and insulin also stimulates the enzyme acetyl-CoA carboxylase and the pathway by which newly formed fatty acids are made into storage fat (triacylglycerol). The stimulation is both rapid, acting via the insulin receptor and its signalling chain, and longer-term, through increased expression of the genes concerned, and hence synthesis of more of the enzymes. That fact, that the synthesis of fat from glucose is stimulated by insulin, has led to dietary claims that we shall discuss shortly.

If glucose can be converted to fat, why cannot fat be converted to glucose? Breakdown of fatty acids leads to acetyl-CoA. Acetyl-CoA cannot be turned into glucose. The starting point for making glucose (the pathway called gluconeogenesis) must be a compound with three carbon atoms – for instance, lactic acid, pyruvic acid, or glycerol. Acetyl-CoA gets consumed in the citric acid cycle before it can make any of these. You could well ask 'Why?'. It doesn't have to be so. Organisms other than animals – plants, bacteria, fungi – have a variation on the citric acid cycle, called the glyoxylate cycle, that enables the carbons from acetyl-CoA to enter the gluconeogenesis pathway. Why don't we have this? That's a philosophical question: presumably it hasn't been important in our evolution to use fat to make glucose. Fatty acids, and their partial oxidation product the ketone bodies, can satisfy much of our metabolic needs.

The Importance of Lipogenesis

The conversion of glucose into fat is stimulated by insulin. So it seems obvious that eating carbohydrates, especially simple sugars, will raise insulin secretion and make us fat. Or so it might seem.

There is no doubt that the pathway for making fat from carbohydrate is important for some animals. Laboratory rats and mice are usually fed a very dull diet in the form of compressed pellets of cereal with little fat. Little wonder, then, that their fat stores, such as they are, are largely made from the pathway of lipogenesis. The trouble is that so much of our early understanding of metabolism was based on studies of laboratory rodents. So there has been an assumption amongst the biochemical community, that has translated to the wider world, that this pathway is how we lay down fat.

People who consume very little fat must also use this pathway. The group in whom this has been carefully studied are patients who cannot take nutrients through the gastrointestinal tract (e.g. because of intestinal surgery), and have to receive their nutrition by vein. Nowadays such patients will receive a mixture of glucose, amino acids, and fat, together with vitamins and nutrients.

But when techniques of intravenous feeding were being developed, during the 1970s and early 1980s, there was no safe way to give fat into a vein, and these patients received their energy from glucose and amino acids. Patients could gain weight on this simple mixture, which seemed good news to the physicians looking after them, as they wanted their patients to build up muscle. Rod King and colleagues at the University of Leeds, UK, carried out detailed studies of such patients. They used an indirect calorimetry apparatus, enabling them to see what was happening to glucose and fat oxidation. After a few days of feeding, the pathway of lipogenesis was activated, and the patients began to lay down fat from their incoming glucose. It was not what the physicians wanted, of course: they wanted the patients to use glucose for energy and amino acids to build up muscles.

In the early 1980s, then, there was a general belief that the pathway of lipogenesis was an important route by which we lay down fat in times of energy excess. But that changed following a series of studies by the group led by Eric Jequiér, Professor of Physiology at the University of Lausanne in Switzerland. Jequiér and his colleagues, including Yves Schutz and Kevin Acheson, a British scientist working in the associated laboratories of the Nestlé company, were amongst world leaders in human calorimetry. They had whole-body human calorimeter chambers, in which people could live whilst their energy expenditure was being measured and information gathered on which fuels the body was using. These experimenters investigated the role of *de novo* lipogenesis (fat synthesis from glucose) in humans. Acheson recruited a group of healthy volunteers and fed them a very high-carbohydrate breakfast: 480 grams (g) of carbohydrate 'in the form of bread, jam, and fruit juice' – lots of rapidly digestible carbohydrates, just the sort we would have expected to raise insulin secretion and turn into fat. The volunteers were then studied in the calorimetry chamber to measure how much fat they laid down from this big carbohydrate load. But they didn't. Over the next 10 hours, the results were as follows: oxidation of 29 g protein, 133 g carbohydrate, and 17 g fat (all these figures are 'net': there may have been both oxidation and synthesis of fat, but if so, the former outweighed the latter). To be clear, the volunteers over this period *oxidised* fat in a net sense; they didn't *make* it. (Even over shorter periods, the experimenters reported, if there were times of net fat synthesis, they were transient.) Knowing the amount of carbohydrate eaten and the amount oxidised, the experimenters could calculate that there was a net gain of nearly 350 g of glycogen.

This went against what many believed about the 'fattening' power of large carbohydrate intakes. As the authors summarised their findings: 'These findings challenge the common perception that conversion of carbohydrate to fat is an important pathway for the retention of dietary energy and for the accumulation of body fat'.

A later study from the group in Lausanne shed light on the physiological role of *de novo* lipogenesis in humans. This time they studied volunteers over a longer period. Initially the volunteers received a low-carbohydrate, low-energy diet and they exercised, so that their glycogen stores were depleted. Then they were given a diet that was rich in carbohydrate, and supplied more energy than their bodies required, for 7 days – 'overfeeding'. By making careful measurements of metabolic balances (intake and oxidation), the experimenters showed that over the first 4 days, the volunteers were refilling their glycogen stores to the tune of about '15 g / kg body weight' – so for a 65 kg person, the average in the study, this amounted to almost 1 kg of glycogen, much more than most of us would have thought possible. But the really interesting finding was that, after about 500 g of glycogen had been accumulated, their bodies began to make fat in a net sense: it became a way for the body to dispose of excess carbohydrate that could not be oxidised and could not be stored as glycogen. By the end of 7 days of over-feeding, the volunteers were converting around 500 g of carbohydrate per day into fat. The results are illustrated in Figure 8.3.

In humans, then, it seems that the role of the pathway of *net* conversion of glucose into fat is not to lay down fat during day-to-day life, but to provide a mechanism for disposal of excess glucose when other avenues – oxidation and glycogen synthesis – are saturated.

But there certainly are important metabolic roles for the pathway of *de novo* lipogenesis, which is operating most of the time, but not creating fat in a *net* sense – fat oxidation still outweighs new fat synthesis. One of these roles concerns regulation of fat oxidation, that I shall come back to shortly.

Amino Acids Are also Intimately Linked with Glucose and Fat Metabolism

Each protein molecule in our bodies is made up of amino acids in a particular order. There are twenty different amino acids making up most proteins – they have been called the 'alphabet of protein structure'. Different proteins have

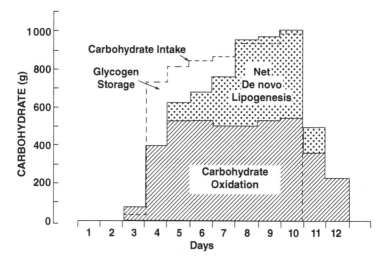

Figure 8.3 Net conversion of carbohydrate to fat when volunteers are over-fed a carbohydrate-rich diet. The figure shows how the dietary carbohydrate was disposed of each day. The over-feeding began on day 4 on this graph and finished on day 10. The blank white area shows conversion of dietary carbohydrate to glycogen; the stippled grey area shows conversion to fat.

different proportions of these amino acids, although it is possible to generalise to some extent. So we can give a typical amino acid composition of the proteins that make up muscles.

But the pattern of amino acids present in blood looks quite different from any protein. Two amino acids, glutamine and alanine, are generally present in greater concentrations than any other. In the 1970s, the source of these amino acids in blood was investigated by Philip Felig and others at Yale University, US. They put plastic tubes, catheters, into veins that carry blood away from muscles and compared the amino acids in those veins with the concentrations entering the muscles (arterial blood), and showed clearly that glutamine and alanine predominate in amino acid release from muscle. And yet, the amino acid composition of muscle proteins did not show any particular predominance of these amino acids.

Alanine is the easier to understand. It is a small amino acid, with a structure similar to pyruvic acid, the half-way product of glucose breakdown – except

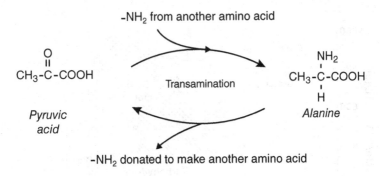

Figure 8.4 Transamination interconverts amino acids and other metabolites.

that it has the 'amino' group (represented -NH$_2$) that pyruvic acid does not. Felig postulated that this alanine leaving muscle was really 'pyruvic acid in disguise'.

Some amino acids are oxidised in muscles, as a source of energy. This applies particularly to a group of three amino acids called the 'branched-chain amino acids' because the chains of carbon atoms making them up are branched. As we have noted, when amino acids are oxidised, their amino group, containing the nitrogen atom, must be transferred to the liver, where the nitrogen is converted to urea for excretion. A common reaction during the breakdown of amino acids is that their amino group is passed to a metabolite that is an acid; what remains is then itself an acid (as these are amino *acids*). This is called transamination (swapping of amino groups) and is shown in Figure 8.4.

So, a large proportion of the alanine leaving muscle is derived from pyruvic acid, i.e. from glycolysis. It is carrying amino-nitrogen to the liver for conversion to urea and excretion. The first step in its metabolism in the liver cell will be a further transamination, taking off its amino group, so leaving pyruvic acid, a 3-carbon molecule that can serve to make new glucose through the pathway of gluconeogenesis. The amino group will make its way into the urea cycle for final excretion as urea. If you refer back to the diagram of the Cori cycle (Figure 6.2), you can add to the transport of lactic acid back to the liver also some pyruvic acid, and some alanine – all fulfilling the same purpose.

Several amino acids, when losing their amino groups by the process of transamination, become metabolites important in carbohydrate and fat metabolism. The names are not important here, but two common amino acids after transamination become compounds that are intermediates in the citric acid cycle. This can be important to keep up flow through the cycle. Some intermediates are always being 'tapped off' and there needs to be a mechanism to top up the intermediates.

Glucose, Fat, and Insulin

A key mediator of the relationships between glucose and fat metabolism is, not surprisingly, insulin. When the glucose concentration in blood rises, typically after eating carbohydrate, then insulin is produced, and shuts off fat mobilisation (breakdown of stored triacylglycerol with release of fatty acids into the blood). This has long been understood (albeit sometimes forgotten), and we looked at it in Chapter 6.

The ability of insulin to shut down fat mobilisation is quite remarkable. This is probably the metabolic process most sensitive to insulin in humans. We had a good illustration from some of our own experiments. We took small blood samples from a catheter placed in one of the tiny veins that you can just see on the abdominal wall that is carrying blood away from the adipose tissue stored there (the 'tummy fat'). We also took blood samples from an artery, representing the blood reaching the adipose tissue: and we looked for differences between them, to show us what the adipose tissue was doing. Here we concentrate on the release of fatty acids (shown in Figure 8.5, as non-esterified fatty acids, or NEFA), representing the process of fat mobilisation.

A group of healthy volunteers came in for experiments after fasting overnight. The volunteers lay still in bed for a couple of hours whilst we drew blood samples. During the first hour, you can see a typical concentration of fatty acids in arterial blood (dark grey, solid circles) at about 500 μmol/l, or 0.5 mmol/l. You can also see where these fatty acids are coming from. The concentration of fatty acids in the little vein leaving the adipose tissue is about 1 000–1 200 μmol/l (1.0–1.2 mmol/l) (light grey, open circles) – this is where they are coming from, before getting mixed into the general circulation. (It's as though we were looking at the exit from the hospital car park at going-home

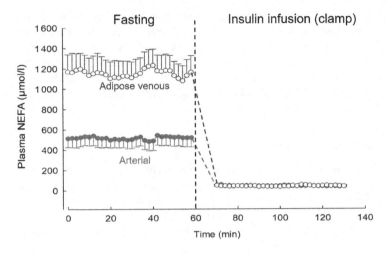

Figure 8.5 Insulin and fatty acid release. Solid circles (dark grey) represent blood in arteries. Open circles (light grey) represent samples taken from the vein draining adipose tissue. An infusion of insulin into the bloodstream was started after 60 minutes, suppressing the release of fatty acids from the adipose tissue depot.

time: cars are pouring out onto the main carriageway, where they are more spread out.) This state remains fairly steady for the first hour.

After 60 minutes, we used a technique called 'glucose clamp'. We wanted to look at the effect of insulin on fatty acid release from adipose tissue. We used a pump to deliver insulin into a vein, raising the concentration of insulin in the bloodstream to the level that would occur after a meal. On its own, that would be a disastrous experiment: insulin would cause the blood glucose concentration to fall and the subject would slip into unconsciousness. The 'glucose clamp' involves also setting up a solution of glucose to infuse into a vein. At the bedside we had a rapid analyser, so that every 2 minutes we could take a small sample of blood, measure the glucose concentration, and then – using a computer programme – adjust the rate at which we pumped in the glucose solution to keep the glucose concentration absolutely constant (hence 'clamped'). You can see what happened to fatty acid release from adipose tissue at 60 minutes when we started the insulin: straight down to zero in a matter of moments (and the arterial level, representing the supply to other tissues, fell close to zero). After a meal, the insulin concentration will rise more gradually, and hence fat mobilisation will take longer to respond – but respond it will. Let nobody say that insulin is the hormone that controls 'blood sugar': it has at least an equally important role in controlling fatty acids.

In recent years we have learned of another side to this relationship between glucose, fatty acids, and insulin. Fatty acids themselves increase insulin secretion (some individual fatty acids more than others). If an experimenter measures the insulin response to a rise in plasma glucose concentration, then repeats the experiment whilst artificially raising the concentration of fatty acids in the bloodstream (for which there are experimental methods available), then the insulin response will be greater. The β-cells of the islets of Langerhans are sensing these fatty acids in some way and adjusting insulin secretion accordingly. This could be seen as an additional mechanism limiting fatty acid release (fat mobilisation) when glucose is available: if for some reason the fatty acid concentration is elevated more than it should be, then more insulin will be produced to shut it down.

The Glucose Fatty-acid Cycle and Other Mechanisms

But we also know of mechanisms that operate within cells to adjust the relative utilisation of glucose and fatty acids according to their availability.

In 1963, four Cambridge metabolic scientists, Philip Randle, Eric Newsholme, Nick Hales, and Peter Garland, published a paper in the medical journal The Lancet entitled 'The glucose fatty-acid cycle: Its role in insulin sensitivity and the metabolic disturbances of diabetes mellitus'. (I will use the hyphenation of the original paper, although I don't think it's logical nowadays.) This paper has been extraordinarily influential. It has been cited (referred to in other scientific papers) over 4 000 times. It does not describe a metabolic cycle in the same way as the cycles we have looked at (for instance the citric acid or Cori cycles): it describes a cycle of regulation.

In this paper, the authors began by describing the relationships between glucose, insulin, and fatty acids, as I have outlined above. But they went further: they added observations on various types of muscle studied in the laboratory, showing that when muscles are supplied with fatty acids, then the rate at which they use glucose decreases – independently of any effect of insulin. It makes perfect physiological sense – it could be seen as a further refinement of the mutual interaction of glucose and fatty acids, such that fuels are used according to their abundance.

If fatty acids can suppress the utilisation of glucose, then we might perhaps think there should be a complementary mechanism, whereby glucose suppresses fatty acid use. And indeed there is.

This is a fascinating story of scientific discovery. Denis McGarry, a British-born biochemist, and his colleague Daniel Foster, working at the University of Texas, were exploring a long-standing observation that if the liver is replete with glycogen, then the oxidation of fatty acids is suppressed. They were looking at the ability of various metabolic products, which might result from glycogen and glucose breakdown, to inhibit fatty acid oxidation. In 1977, they discovered that the metabolite responsible is malonyl-CoA. (To recap, acetyl-CoA, with two carbon atoms in its acetyl group, is combined with carbon dioxide by the enzyme acetyl-CoA carboxylase to make malonyl-CoA with three carbon atoms, in the pathway of lipogenesis – fat synthesis.) This is an extremely elegant piece of metabolic regulation. When there is plenty of carbohydrate around, insulin levels will be high, and some glucose diverted into synthesis of fatty acids. As fatty acid synthesis is increased, so the concentration of malonyl-CoA in the cell will increase. As the concentration of malonyl-CoA rises, so it inhibits fatty acid oxidation – since the body doesn't need to oxidise fatty acids when there is plenty of glucose available. Malonyl-CoA does this by inhibiting the transport of fatty acids into mitochondria for oxidation (the process involving carnitine, discussed in Chapter 5), so that they are likely to be converted into storage fat such as triacylglycerol.

What we have learned since, from further work by Denis McGarry as well as other biochemists such as Victor Zammit, working initially at the Hannah Research Institute in Scotland, latterly at the University of Warwick, is that this mechanism is not confined to the liver. Only liver and adipose tissue have the pathway to make fatty acids from acetyl-CoA – they have the enzyme fatty acid synthase, whereas other tissues do not. But if we take skeletal muscle as an example, it cannot make fatty acids – it has no need to – but it does have a version of the enzyme acetyl-CoA carboxylase that makes malonyl-CoA. Why should a tissue that cannot make fatty acids, make malonyl-CoA? The only possible explanation is that malonyl-CoA is produced simply to regulate fatty acid oxidation.

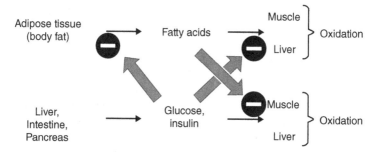

Figure 8.6 Metabolic interactions between glucose (and insulin) and fatty acids. The interactions shown are all 'inhibitory' – e.g. increased availability of glucose (and insulin) reduces release of fatty acids from adipose tissue; glucose and fatty acids mutually reduce the oxidation of each other.

When we looked at muscle metabolism during exercise in the last chapter, I noted that there are observations suggesting that when muscles are working hard, they cannot oxidise fatty acids at a high rate, even if the supply of fatty acids through the blood appears adequate. There is evidence that a high rate of glucose oxidation in muscle during exercise generates malonyl-CoA as a side-process, and that this stops fatty acids being oxidised at a high rate. Because this mechanism is a complement to the glucose fatty-acid cycle, in which fatty acid availability reduces glucose oxidation, it has sometimes been called the 'Reverse glucose fatty-acid cycle'.

You can see how these two regulatory mechanisms work in Figure 8.6.

Longer-term Relationships between Carbohydrate, Fat, and Amino Acid Metabolism

The mechanisms described above linking the metabolic fates of the three major nutrients all operate in the relatively short term – they would affect metabolism in the period after a meal, for instance. But there are also mechanisms that operate over longer timescales. Suppose, for instance, that someone changes from a diet rich in carbohydrate to a diet rich in fat or protein. Our cells have mechanisms that sense the availability of nutrients and adjust the expression of the genes to deal with them (that is, regulate the amount of enzymes or other proteins made from those particular genes). As we saw when we looked at hormone action, such changes take several hours or perhaps days to come into effect.

For instance, there are many genes whose expression is regulated by insulin. These include genes coding for enzymes that will help to dispose of the extra glucose, and also enzymes that help convert any spare glucose to fats, and that help to store away both glucose and fatty acids. Glucose availability also acts (perhaps via a metabolic product of glucose – this is not clear) to regulate gene expression more directly, by increasing the activity of a transcription factor called the carbohydrate response element binding protein (ChREBP). A transcription factor is a protein that can bind to a specific stretch of DNA and increase, or decrease, the expression of a particular gene, thus regulating the amount of the respective enzyme or other protein made in the cell. ChREBP activity, like insulin, increases expression of enzymes that will dispose of carbohydrate and store fat. There are similar mechanisms regulating directly the enzymes of fat storage and amino acid metabolism.

Putting This into Perspective: Metabolic Interactions and Daily Life

I have emphasised that glucose, fatty acid, and amino acid metabolism are intimately connected. You cannot consider one without the others. We must also remember that all fuels – alcohol, amino acids, carbohydrates, and fats – feed (via acetyl-CoA) into the same final common pathway for oxidation, the citric acid cycle. That cycle has finite capacity – if one fuel is being oxidised, it is likely that another is being spared.

In the last chapter, when discussing physical activity, I introduced the idea that some types of exercise might truly be described as 'fat burning'. That would apply, for instance, to exercise at low to moderate intensity, especially prolonged exercise, and necessarily it would apply to exercise carried out in the fasting state. One therefore sees 'fat burning exercise' promoted, on a regular basis, as the type of exercise to concentrate upon if one is interested in losing weight.

But can that be so? Suppose one does 'carbohydrate-burning' exercise. That might mean exercise at a higher intensity and perhaps shorter duration – or exercise after a carbohydrate-rich meal. Will that *not* deplete the fat stores? To suggest not is to fail to grasp how the body's fuels work together. I will explain how I see this, pulling together discussions from earlier chapters. I go out and work out at a high intensity which relies mainly on my glycogen stores. I don't burn much fat. Next time I eat, I am in a carbohydrate-depleted state. Dietary carbohydrate goes to replenish my glycogen stores: less glucose is available for metabolism by other routes, fat oxidation is less inhibited, and I end up dipping into my fat stores sooner than I might have if my glycogen stores had been full. Another day I go out and jog for several hours at a slow pace, using the same amount of energy overall as on the previous occasion, but this time burning mainly fat. Now when I next eat, my glycogen stores are relatively intact, glucose and insulin are more available and suppress mobilisation from my fat stores and also (through the malonyl-CoA mechanism) reduce fat oxidation. Personally, having looked at these mechanisms, and reviewed the relevant experimental data, I fail to see that – at the end of the day - I will lose more of my fat stores with one type of exercise than another. It's the energy expended that matters, not the immediate fuel for oxidation.

So we come towards the end of our tour of human metabolism and how it operates to keep us going in our daily lives, with no conscious intervention from us. But sometimes things can go awry, and for completeness we will next have a look at some metabolic disorders.

9 Metabolic Disorders

Metabolism In and Out of Balance

A large part of this book has been spent examining how human metabolism can adjust to various conditions, some quite extreme, and yet the whole body remain perfectly healthy. But, just as with any complex piece of machinery, things can go wrong. Disorders of metabolism may underlie (or be associated with) many common diseases, especially chronic diseases such as diabetes, cardiovascular disease, and cancer.

Inherited and Acquired Metabolic Disorders

Metabolism depends upon the actions of hundreds, or probably thousands, of proteins, all working perfectly in unison. Each of these proteins has a sequence of amino acids that is specified by the gene that encodes it. But occasionally changes occur in genes that alter the sequence, or number, of amino acids in proteins and affect their function. If that protein is an enzyme involved in metabolism, or one of the many proteins that affect the rate of metabolic reactions (e.g. the receptor for a hormone), then a metabolic pathway may not function optimally. Many such genetic alterations, or mutations, are handed down in families. (Some arise each time a new person is formed.) Many of these will have very small effects that can only be detected by sophisticated testing, if at all. But just a few have effects that are very major. These mutations lie behind the so-called inherited metabolic disorders.

Other metabolic conditions, though, may be the result of environmental factors, a broad term which would include lifestyle and family background. An obvious example is that obesity, the accumulation of adipose tissue to the extent that health is threatened, involves alterations in many metabolic pathways, and some at least of these will underlie the metabolic complications of obesity – for instance, increased risk of developing type 2 diabetes. These conditions are generally referred to as 'acquired'. Nevertheless, although this appears a simple dichotomy, there are grey areas. For instance, there are multiple genetic influences that will affect someone's propensity to become obese.

Inherited Disorders of Metabolism: Different Patterns of Inheritance

In all our cells other than sperm and eggs, we have two copies of each gene (one inherited from each parent). Some genetic mutations affect the function of a protein – for instance an enzyme – so severely that it has no activity. It may be that the other copy of the gene, inherited from the other parent, codes for a protein with normal activity, and that this may be sufficient to keep the pathway active. In that case the person will have normal metabolic function in the pathway but will be a 'carrier' of the mutation, which may be passed on to future generations. If by unlucky chance a carrier were to produce offspring with another carrier of a mutation in that gene, then on average one in four of their offspring would have two copies of the mutation, and the problem would be evident. Such disorders are called 'recessive' as they are only manifest when both copies of the gene are affected. More rarely, a dysfunctional gene can put the whole system out of kilter, so that only one copy is needed for the problem to appear: this is known as a dominant mutation. (An example would be Huntington's disease, in which a mutated gene produces a disease-causing protein.) More common than that are sex-linked mutations. Males carry one copy each of the sex chromosomes, called X and Y, whereas females have two X chromosomes. There are many genes affecting metabolic pathways on the X chromosome. If one of these is defective, then males will always display the problem because they only have one X chromosome, whereas females are likely to be spared as they will probably have one 'good' copy. An example is deficiency of the enzyme glucose-6-phosphate dehydrogenase, an enzyme involved in glucose metabolism that generates 'reducing power' (or hydrogen atoms, {H} in the language of Chapter 5), and is especially important in red blood cells. The gene for this enzyme is on the X-chromosome. Boys carrying a mutation in the enzyme are likely to display symptoms (breakdown of red blood cells, and hence anaemia, usually only in the presence of other stimuli), whereas a girl with one affected gene is less likely to show symptoms.

Metabolic disorders caused by mutations inherited in these ways are described as 'Mendelian', after Gregor Mendel, the Austrian friar (living in what is now the Czech Republic) whose studies of plant reproduction led, later, to the concept of genes.

But there are very many metabolic conditions in which a large number of genes each has a small effect. These are described as polygenic. Obesity is one such condition: from very large samples, it is possible to see influences from something like 100 different genes, but in each case the influence is only tiny.

Disorders of Metabolism Inherited in a Mendelian Fashion

Many diseases caused by a single gene are severe, and often manifest in young children. They are often referred to as 'inborn errors of metabolism'. In some cases, if the problem is recognised early enough, it may be possible to mitigate the effects, e.g. by prescribing a particular diet. An example is phenylketonuria. This is caused by a defect in the gene that codes for the enzyme phenylalanine hydroxylase. Phenylalanine is one of the amino acids that make up proteins. It is broken down by a metabolic pathway that begins with this enzyme. If the enzyme is deficient, phenylalanine accumulates in blood, and causes damage to the central nervous system; some by-products are excreted in the urine (hence the name of the disease). It is standard practice now to screen newborns by measuring the phenylalanine concentration in a tiny drop of blood. If the condition is detected, that individual will need to live on a diet very low in phenylalanine for the rest of their life. But in other conditions, there may be no adequate treatment, and the affected child may die early. Mutations causing less severe metabolic impairments many become manifest later in life, and be compatible with normal longevity.

There are databases of these metabolic disorders inherited in a Mendelian fashion. Online Mendelian Inheritance in Man (OMIM) is a free, online database (© Johns Hopkins University), and such disorders are often referred to by their OMIM catalogue number. Scriver's *The Online Metabolic & Molecular Bases of Inherited Disease* is a commercial catalogue.

There is a very large number of metabolic diseases caused by inheritance of a genetic mutation. They include disorders of carbohydrate, fat, and amino acid metabolism (of which phenylketonuria is the most common). To give a few examples: in carbohydrate metabolism, there is a large group of conditions called Glycogen Storage Diseases. These may be caused by defects in almost any of the enzymes concerned with glycogen storage and breakdown. They are mostly inherited in an autosomal recessive fashion, meaning that the gene is not on a sex chromosome (autosomal), so the incidence is usually the same for males and females, and that a person must have two defective copies of the gene to display symptoms (recessive). The effect on patients is usually related to difficulties in maintaining blood glucose concentrations, or in exercising. The overall prevalence of glycogen storage diseases is around 1 in 20 000 births. The most common form is known as glycogen storage disease type 1a, or Von Gierke disease after the physician who first described it. This results from a defect in the enzyme glucose-6-phosphatase, which converts glucose 6-phosphate (which may come from glycogen breakdown) to glucose in the liver. Therefore, patients with this condition cannot derive blood glucose directly from their liver glycogen, and it is usually detected in the first year of life because of an enlarged liver, and a tendency to hypoglycaemia (low blood glucose, which may in turn cause seizures). It can be managed by feeding a diet with long-chain polysaccharides (such as corn starch) to provide a slow release of glucose, and many patients live well into adulthood, and may themselves become parents.

In fat metabolism, there are many inherited conditions in which the ability to oxidise fatty acids is impaired because of lack of a relevant enzyme function. These conditions may become manifest early in life as a difficulty in maintaining blood glucose concentration: as we have seen, when the diet is mainly fat-based (milk), the brain will require either glucose or ketone bodies to be made in the liver. Gluconeogenesis requires energy derived from oxidation of fatty acids; ketone bodies are derived directly from fatty acid oxidation. An example would be a defect in the enzyme very long-chain acyl-CoA dehydrogenase, which is the first step in the oxidation of fatty acids (other than those with medium or short carbon chains). This can manifest in various ways. Severe forms are manifest as heart problems in infancy, as the heart requires energy from oxidation of fatty acids. More commonly, perhaps because the enzyme activity is not entirely lost, it is diagnosed in adult life because of muscle problems brought on by exercise. Dietary management will include provision of carbohydrate as an energy source, and restriction of the amount of long-chain fatty acids (all the common dietary fatty acids) in the diet: they may be substituted with fatty acids of shorter carbon chain-length in the form usually called medium-chain triacylglycerols. There are also diseases relating to inability to oxidise more complex lipids, and often these impact upon nervous system function.

Perhaps the most common inherited disorder of fat metabolism relates to a pathway that we have not considered in this book – the ability of cells to take up cholesterol, and thus remove it from the blood. This occurs through a protein called the LDL receptor (LDL, low-density lipoprotein, often called 'bad cholesterol', is the form in which most blood cholesterol is found). People with a mutation in the LDL receptor have high levels of cholesterol in the blood and – if the condition is not treated – are strongly at risk of heart attack (myocardial infarction) at an early age. In this case, normal function requires two functional copies of the gene, so the condition, called Familial Hypercholesterolaemia, is usually heterozygous – meaning the person has only one mutated gene, and one normal. Around 1 in 500 people worldwide have this condition. Fortunately, nowadays, provided the condition is detected in good time, it can be treated with a statin drug to lower blood cholesterol, and the patient can expect normal longevity.

Polygenic and Acquired Metabolic Disorders: A Grey Area

Diseases caused by mutations in single genes, and inherited in Mendelian fashion, are all relatively rare. Other metabolic conditions that are much more common may have partly genetic and partly environmental (or behavioural) causes: and all those influences may be very difficult to disentangle. We will look briefly at the condition of obesity, defined as an excessive accumulation of fat in the body. (It may be debatable whether to call obesity a metabolic condition. Certainly many features of metabolism are disturbed in obesity. But it will illustrate the point.)

Obesity is sometimes characterised as a 'lifestyle condition', implying that the sufferer has some choice in the matter. But that fails to reflect the very strong inherited pattern of obesity. At one time, it was considered that the familial pattern of obesity reflected family habits, such as ways of preparing food ('it's the frying pan that's inherited'). A series of studies from the 1980s onwards has shown that this is a small component. Studies of identical (monozygotic) twins (with almost identical genes), who were separated at birth and adopted into different households, show that the pattern of body weight (thin or over-weight) is much more strongly related to the birth family than to the family in which someone grew up. Numerical estimates of the inheritance of obesity suggest that around two thirds of the variation seen in adult fatness or thinness is down to genetics. The inheritance is higher when children are studied (genes affect them more than adults, in whom environmental influences have a greater effect). In a study of twins aged 7 and 10 years in the UK, published in 2008, the figure for heritability of fatness was 0.7 (or 70%); the equivalent figure for the influence of 'shared environment' was more like 0.2. This means that when we look at a group of children of that age, we will see variation in their fatness. Of that variation, a major part is down to genes, and only a small part of that variation is down to other factors such as cooking habits in the family.

And yet, attempts to pin down which genes are responsible have proved difficult. A few genes have been identified that underly a proportion (a few percent typically) of cases of extreme obesity, especially in children: these genes are almost all in the pathways that regulate appetite in the brain. Studies in which all the human genes (the human genome) were scanned, looking for links with obesity, have led to identification of several hundred genetic loci – positions on the DNA – that can influence body weight. But the influence of each may be very, very small. In a paper published in 2015 it was estimated that '97 loci have been identified as accounting for about 2.7% of variation in body mass index [a commonly used measure of leanness or fatness]'. In addition, these studies can be difficult to interpret in terms of metabolism, as very often the investigators cannot say what the function of the gene con-cerned is – if, indeed, a gene is identified. In many cases a position in the DNA is located but not necessarily even within a gene.

This all leads to the conclusion that the classic distinction between 'inherited' and 'acquired' metabolic disorders is a gross oversimplification. We will see this illustrated when we consider one of the most common disorders of metabolism, diabetes.

Diabetes: A Widespread Disorder of Metabolism

Just to be clear at the outset, the term 'diabetes' covers a variety of conditions. One, strictly called *diabetes insipidus*, has nothing to do with metabolism: it is a disorder of the hormonal system that regulates urine production, resulting in patients producing too much urine, which is of necessity dilute and watery or 'insipid'. In contrast, the group of conditions called *diabetes mellitus* are very much metabolic disorders. *Mellitus*, from the Greek word for honey, relates to the fact that the urine of people with this condition, whilst also produced in excess, tastes sweet (physicians in days gone by would taste the urine). This is because it contains glucose, which normal urine does not.

Diabetes mellitus (which I simply refer to as diabetes here) is not a single disease. There are two major forms, called now type 1 and type 2, although within each of these there are multiple sub-types. But they have one thing in common. Diabetes mellitus always results from an insufficient action of the hormone insulin. Because the condition was first recognised through the sugar in the urine, and because diagnostic tests rely on finding too much glucose in the blood, it is common to think of diabetes as a disorder of carbohydrate metabolism. However, as we have seen throughout this book, insulin regulates fat and amino acid metabolism also, and these are also affected.

Insulin, as we have seen, is a hormone which is a protein, produced in the β-cells of the pancreatic islets of Langerhans (see Figure 4.1). In some people, the body's immune system starts to attack its own tissues – this is 'autoimmune disease'. If the attack is on the pancreatic β-cells, they may be destroyed and therefore unable to produce insulin. This brings about a state of absolute insulin deficiency. It may be impossible to measure any insulin in a blood sample. That is the situation in type 1 diabetes. It usually comes on early in life, although sometimes in adulthood. The trigger that causes the immune system to attack the β-cells is unknown. It is a serious condition and must be treated. The only possible treatment is to replace the missing insulin, by injection. Fortunately, nowadays insulin identical to human insulin can be made using recombinant-DNA techniques – putting the human insulin gene into the DNA of bacteria, which can be grown in big tanks, and the insulin harvested and purified. In former days, insulin for injection was prepared from the pancreas of slaughtered cows or pigs. It might contain impurities, and because it was not identical to human insulin, the patient might develop antibodies that made it less effective.

Type 1 diabetes has an inherited component, but it's not especially strong: there is a risk of less than 10% of developing the condition for a child of a parent with type 1 diabetes. The overall lifetime risk of developing type 1 diabetes varies greatly by country and geographical region, but overall is around one in 250 people.

In the absence of insulin, all those metabolic processes that we have seen are regulated by insulin will operate in an unregulated way. The liver will produce glucose, initially by breaking down glycogen, then by increased gluconeogenesis: but muscles and other tissues will be unable to use glucose because of lack of insulin. So glucose will accumulate in the blood: the 'hallmark' of diabetes. When the glucose concentration in blood, normally about 5 mmol/l, increases beyond a certain point (around 9 mmol/l, but it varies from person to person), the kidneys can no longer keep up, and glucose is lost in the urine. The presence of glucose in the urine draws water with it, so increased urine production is a feature. Loss of glucose in the urine implies loss of energy from the body, and the sufferer will lose weight. But equally dramatic, although less obvious, changes occur in fat and amino acid metabolism. Fat mobilisation (breakdown of the triacylglycerol in fat cells, releasing fatty acids) is unrestrained: fatty acids accumulate in blood, and oxidation of fatty acids in the liver is also unrestrained, so ketone bodies are formed at a high rate. The accumulation of fatty acids and ketone bodies in blood makes the blood acidic, and this is one reason for the seriousness of this condition, called diabetic ketoacidosis (we looked at it also in connection with starvation, Chapter 7). Proteins will also break down as insulin's normal protein-building effect is absent. The whole metabolic picture is one of 'catabolism' (breakdown of complex molecules and tissues). As noted earlier, this serious metabolism condition can only be treated by replacement of insulin (Figure 9.1).

Type 2 diabetes is much more common than type 1 diabetes (around 80% of cases of diabetes mellitus are type 2). The mechanism is different. It is strongly associated with obesity – although thin people can also develop it, perhaps as a result of genetics. One widely accepted theory about its development is that, as fat accumulates because of an energy surplus, the fat cells can no longer cope, and fat (triacylglycerol and other lipids) ends up in tissues where it should not be stored, including liver, muscles, and the pancreas. Accumulation of triacylglycerol in tissues somehow reduces their ability to respond to insulin – the condition known as insulin resistance. Accumulation of triacylglycerol in the pancreas may reduce the ability of the β-cells to secrete insulin. As fat accumulates, the pancreas needs to produce more

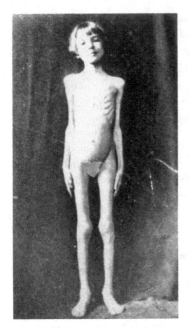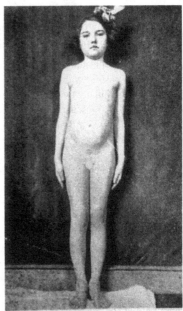

Figure 9.1 A sufferer from type 1 diabetes in the very early days of insulin treatment, before (left) and after (right) treatment with insulin.

insulin to counteract the insulin resistance, but at some point this ability fails, and there is a lack of the necessary insulin – although the concentration of insulin, measured in blood, may not be particularly low. Then the metabolic picture will be as described for type 1 diabetes, although generally less severe – diabetic ketoacidosis can occur in type 2 diabetes, but is not common.

However, equally severe in both type 1 and type 2 diabetes is the development of complications, related to the high blood glucose concentration, affecting many organs and tissues including eyes, kidneys, nerves, and the cardiovascular system. For that reason, treatment is essential to maintain health and normal longevity. Treatment of type 2 diabetes has changed dramatically in the past couple of decades. It is now recognised that rapid and significant loss of weight can reverse the diabetes, especially early in the disease. This may be achieved by 'bariatric surgery' – surgery to the gastro-intestinal tract to limit the ability to take in and absorb food, and perhaps with a hormonal effect on appetite; or by very strict dieting, typically beginning with a very low-calorie diet of perhaps 3–4 MJ/day (say 1 000 kcal/day) for 12 weeks. Beyond that, medicines are needed. The traditional treatment for type 2 diabetes was a drug of the sulfonylurea class: these stimulate insulin secretion from the pancreatic β-cells. Now we have additional medicines including those that improve insulin resistance, a new group acting on hormone systems in the gut that reduce appetite and also stimulate insulin secretion, and most recently drugs that act on the kidneys to cause more glucose to be excreted in urine – thus removing glucose from the blood, and energy from the body.

Cardiovascular Disease and Metabolism

Cardiovascular disease refers to diseases of the heart and the blood vessels. It most commonly appears as a heart attack (myocardial infarction), when blood supply to the heart muscle is blocked, or stroke, when blood supply to part of the brain is blocked (less commonly in Western societies, stroke can also result from a bleed into the brain). There is also disease of the arteries in the limbs, peripheral arterial disease, which can lead to tissue death and ultimately may require amputation of a limb. Underlying all these conditions is the process called atherosclerosis – the build-up of fatty lesions, called plaques, in the walls of blood vessels, especially arteries. Cardiovascular disease is a major cause of death. In those below 70 years of age, the World Health Organization reports that cardiovascular disease accounts for 38% of deaths from non-communicable disease, compared with 27% for deaths from cancer, worldwide. (Non-communicable diseases are those not involving infection.) These figures are changing, however, as the incidence of cardiovascular disease decreases in higher-income countries, where cancer is now a greater cause of death.

Atherosclerosis is a complex process involving inflammation of the artery wall, build-up of various cells and an increase in the muscle cells that line arteries, and the accumulation of lipids in the plaque. High blood pressure increases the risk of developing atherosclerosis. It is in the accumulation of lipid that metabolism is most closely involved. Much of this lipid is cholesterol, and it is derived from cholesterol in the blood in the form of low-density lipoprotein, LDL (mentioned earlier in connection with the condition familial hypercholesterolaemia). The higher the concentration of cholesterol in LDL in the blood, the more it is likely to penetrate the arterial wall and begin to accumulate. The concentration of LDL-cholesterol in the blood is determined by both production (from the liver) and removal (into all tissues). The latter especially is strongly genetically determined, as described earlier for familial hypercholesterolaemia, but production from the liver is affected by a number of metabolic processes, including the amount of fat stored in the liver.

The discovery of the mechanisms by which cholesterol is removed from the bloodstream led directly to a treatment for high cholesterol levels, the statin drugs. These inhibit cholesterol synthesis in cells (the pathway, like synthesis of fatty acids, lipogenesis, begins with acetyl-CoA). Inhibition of cholesterol synthesis leads the cell to take up more cholesterol. This happens especially in the liver, and the cholesterol can then be excreted – lost from the body.

To add a further complication, cholesterol can be removed from tissues by another process, called reverse cholesterol transport, and taken back to the liver from where it can be excreted in bile. This process, which involves another form of cholesterol in blood called high-density lipoprotein (HDL)-cholesterol, is strongly related to levels of triacylglycerol in the blood. Insulin resistance and obesity are associated with raised blood levels of triacylglycerol, and lower levels of HDL-cholesterol, which means that more cholesterol stays in the tissues, including artery walls, and causes damage. Drugs have been developed that target this process, increasing levels of HDL-cholesterol in blood, but so far these have not been found to be clinically useful. Beyond that, the topic of cholesterol metabolism is complex and outside the scope of this book.

Cancer and Metabolism

A cell becomes cancerous when a change in its DNA leads it to be able to divide and spread without the normal limits on these processes. That is not primarily a metabolic phenomenon, although there are strong links between obesity and risk of a number of types of cancer including bowel, breast, and prostate cancer. Being obese is said to be the biggest modifiable risk for cancer after smoking. (Non-modifiable risk factors include age and genetics.)

But once a cell has become cancerous, its metabolism changes. This was first noted by the German biochemist Otto Warburg, mentor to Hans Krebs. He found that tumours, when studied in the laboratory, used glucose at high rates, but largely by the pathway of glycolysis, releasing lactic acid, rather than oxidising the glucose completely in the citric acid cycle. This occurred despite normal oxygen availability, and indeed the tumours also used oxygen. This is known now as the Warburg effect, and the process has been called aerobic glycolysis (glycolysis occurring in the presence of plenty of oxygen). It is thought that the benefit to the tumour cell may be that several pathways important for making cellular components feed off intermediates in the pathway of glycolysis: one example is the pentose-phosphate pathway, which starts with glucose 6-phosphate and produces the sugar ribose needed for DNA and RNA synthesis, and reducing power for making other cellular components such as lipids. Although many attempts have been made to target this metabolic change in order to deprive cancer cells of energy, no clinical treatments have arisen as yet.

The fact that tumour cells use glucose at a high rate has, though, led to advances in cancer diagnosis. A highly radioactive compound closely related to glucose is called fluorodeoxyglucose – it is 'labelled' with a radioactive isotope of fluorine, ^{18}F. The 'deoxy' part makes a glucose molecule that is taken up into cells, then stays there. So, the patient is given a dose of fluorodeoxyglucose, which is taken up especially into tumours because of their high rate of glucose uptake, and then using an external camera to visualise the radioactivity, the tumours can be located. This is known as positron-emission tomography (PET).

More recently, another aspect of metabolism in tumour cells has attracted attention: a high rate of synthesis of fatty acids, by the pathway of *de novo* lipogenesis. This would be facilitated by the production of reducing power from the pentose phosphate pathway, mentioned above. It is thought that the cancer cell needs additional lipids to increase in size and divide. Again, attempts have been made to target this process, and trials are under way with a number of drugs.

One unexpected finding concerns metformin, a drug used to treat type 2 diabetes, in common use since the 1960s. Several retrospective analyses of patients taking metformin have shown a lower cancer incidence than in people not taking it. Metformin is now being investigated as a potential adjuvant in cancer treatment. It has complex effects on metabolism, but one of these is a suppression of lipogenesis. Maybe that relates to its anti-cancer properties.

Metabolic Disorders: Conclusions

The field of metabolic disease is a vast one and we have just skimmed over the surface here. But I hope the message is clear, that disturbances in metabolism underlie many rare and common diseases, and that the understanding of metabolism that has developed over the past century or so places physicians in a good position to understand these diseases and develop treatments.

As we have seen, some disorders of metabolism are directly caused by mutations in genes coding for proteins involved in metabolism. There is little we can do to avoid these, but new treatments are on the way, with some recent developments in gene therapy, whereby a 'good' copy of the defective gene can be introduced to the body. Other diseases involve changes in metabolism and often relate to factors in our environment and in our behaviour. A very large group of adverse metabolic conditions is related to being overweight or obese and being too sedentary. In those cases, anything we can do to change that situation – losing weight and/or increasing levels of physical activity – is likely to change our metabolism for the better.

Concluding Remarks: Human Metabolism in Context

Many years ago now, I spent three busy years studying biochemistry. After my first degree, I researched for three years for my PhD, studying a new treatment for diabetes called metformin – now an old drug, but still widely used, and a first line of treatment for many patients. (We still don't really know how it works.) Then I worked for about half my career studying metabolic responses to trauma – of the physical kind, not the mental. This involved many studies of patients in hospital with injuries or following major operations. It was difficult work – nobody sets out to be injured and so there is no standardisation of feeding state, alcohol intake, time of day, or any of the other factors one would normally control in metabolic experiments; not even a standard form of injury. This research gave me a very clear view of the mechanisms that integrate human metabolism under stress. But it wasn't until I moved to the University of Oxford, about the middle of my career, and started studying metabolism in healthier people, that I understood that our daily lives involve much more subtle changes in metabolic pathways, brought about less by the nervous system and much more by hormones, especially insulin.

So the question arises, whether it is possible to condense the knowledge gained from a lifetime's varied work on human metabolism into a short book for the non-scientist. Only you can judge whether I have succeeded. Of course, one important way to do this has been to remove detail. I could have written a chapter on the enzymes that control the storage of fat in our adipose tissue. But that would have risked the reader missing the wood for the trees. Here I have tried to convey an overall sense of the major metabolic pathways that underlie our daily lives, and of how they are regulated and coordinated.

I have deliberately not strayed too much into the field of obesity, although I am sure that many readers will wish that I had done so. That would have required too many additional chapters. If that was your interest when you started reading this book, then at least I hope that you have gained sufficient knowledge of metabolism to be able to interpret some of the things you will read in the popular press. (And the good news is that a new addition to the series, *Understanding Obesity*, written by my Oxford colleague Professor Stanley Ulijaszek, is on its way.)

So, what should you take away from this book, provided that you are not completely baffled? I would suggest that a key message is that the different nutrients interact within us, and that the citric acid cycle is a final common pathway for their ultimate breakdown. That understanding will immediately tell you that we cannot consider nutrients in isolation. If I cut down on one, something else must make up the deficit: if I take too much of one, others will also be in surplus. I hope also to have been able to explain something of the workings of hormones – often a black box to the outsider. For those who love exercise, I hope you will also have learned something about the metabolic changes that accompany physical activity, and how you might prepare for them. I myself have gained an enormous respect for the generations of metabolic scientists who provided the foundations of our modern understanding of human metabolism, working with tools that seem unsophisticated by present standards.

Our metabolism begins (arguably) very soon after the moment an egg is fertilised by a sperm. It develops through many stages, adapting to our lifestyle as we go from neonate to weanling, to adolescent and adult, and finally into old age. Although it has been my profession to study much of this, I can honestly say that for the most part I really haven't needed to think about my own changing metabolism. I think that probably sums up just how wonderful human metabolism really is.

Summary of Common Misunderstandings

Metabolism is about whether you are fat or thin. Metabolism underlies all aspects of our daily lives. There's a lot more to it than body weight.

Fat is bad for you. The body stores fat as a long-term, but dynamic, energy reserve. People who lack body fat because of a genetic condition are not healthy. That said, too much fat in the body is not good for health either. Fat in the diet is another matter. There are two different issues – the type of fat (whether saturated or unsaturated) and the amount. We cannot live without eating some fat. And there are very good reasons why we have evolved to store our long-term energy reserve as fat rather than carbohydrate or protein.

Fat is good for you. The same applies. Small amounts of some types of fat (certain polyunsaturated fatty acids) are essential for life, but too much fat of any sort adds to energy intake.

Sugars are poisons. That suggestion has been made very strongly by, e.g. Robert Lustig, a paediatric endocrinologist at the University of California at San Francisco, who argues in a much-viewed YouTube video that a high-sugar diet is metabolically equivalent to a high-fat diet, and equally bad for you. Your brain uses sugar (the sugar called glucose) all the time and would fail if glucose were not supplied (other than in starvation, when it can use other fuels). Too much sugar in the diet may be bad, but that's mainly because it adds calories.

Lactate is a metabolic poison and makes your muscles hurt when you exercise. Lactic acid, or lactate, is a normal part of the metabolic breakdown of glucose. It may accumulate in the muscles and blood during strenuous exercise, but that is part of a metabolic mechanism that allows you to exercise harder than you otherwise could. Lactic acid is also a means of preserving carbohydrate stores in lean times.

Hormones are what make you moody. Hormones are signals that govern much of our lives. Some regulate metabolism during normal daily life (insulin is a good example). Adrenaline is a hormone involved in stressful situations (exercise, or 'fight or flight'). And the way hormones work is absolutely remarkable. Tiny concentrations of hormones in the blood can regulate major metabolic process.

Ketone bodies (chemicals that accumulate in the blood in some conditions, causing the state called ketosis) are (1) toxic – a common medical view, or (2) the key to successful slimming (current popular view). Ketone bodies are a normal part of the breakdown of body fat, and play an important role in coordinating metabolism, and especially as a fuel during starvation. In medical practice, ketone body accumulation in someone with diabetes can signal a deteriorating, and potentially lethal, metabolic situation. Ketosis is also a feature of starvation as the liver produces ketone bodies as a fuel for the brain – this is an adaptation that allows survival in the absence of dietary carbohydrate intake. Those taking a very low carbohydrate diet to aid weight loss will experience some ketosis, but this merely shows that the body is in a state of negative energy balance.

If I exercise first thing in the morning, I will burn off more fat. The concept of 'fat-burning exercise' is popular. It refers to exercise in a fasted state (e.g. before breakfast), or exercise at a low intensity for a long period. In these situations, yes, it is true that the muscles will mainly use fat as a fuel. But the close links between carbohydrate and fat metabolism mean that, ultimately, it is the 'calories burned' that matter, not the immediate fuel for the muscles.

A low-carbohydrate diet is the key to slimming as carbohydrates stimulate insulin secretion and insulin makes us lay down fat. This view has been popularised by a number of writers about diet. There is no doubt that some people find that restriction of dietary carbohydrate helps them lose weight, but the same is also true of restriction of fat intake. The story about insulin causing fat to be laid down is a pseudo-metabolic view that fails to appreciate the wonderful and intimate connections between all the nutrients in the course of metabolism.

References

Preface

My student textbook referred to here is Frayn, K. N. & Evans, R. D. (2019). *Human Metabolism: A Regulatory Perspective*, 4th edn. Oxford: Wiley Blackwell.

Chapter 1

On the history of studies in human metabolism: Kleiber, M. (1961). *The Fire of Life: An Introduction to Animal Energetics*. New York: Wiley; McKie, D. (1990). *Antoine Lavoisier: Scientist, Economist, Social Reformer*. New York: Da Capo Press; Noble, D. (2008). Claude Bernard, the first systems biologist, and the future of physiology. *Exp Physiol* 93: 16–26.

On Professor Sir Hans Krebs: Hans Krebs – Facts www.nobelprize.org/prizes/ medicine/1953/krebs/facts/ (on this website, you can read more about Hans Krebs and his discoveries in metabolism); Krebs, H. A. (1967). The making of a scientist. *Nature* 215: 1441–1445. (Hans Krebs, perhaps the most widely known metabolic scientist, explains how his receipt of the Nobel Prize reflected fortunate chances during his earlier years); Whitehead, D. (2010). Oh to be in Oxford now that Krebs is there…! *The Biochemist* 32: 54–55. (David Whitehead reflects on a time of metabolic discoveries in Oxford – and featuring an often-reproduced photo of Hans Krebs astride a moped – perhaps the original Krebs cycle?)

Chapter 2

On human liver glycogen: Nilsson, L. H. & Hultman, E. (1973). Liver glycogen in man – the effect of total starvation or a carbohydrate-poor diet followed by carbohydrate refeeding. *Scand J Clin Lab Invest* 32: 325–330.

On more detailed background reading: Frayn, K. N. & Evans, R. D. (2019). *Human Metabolism: A Regulatory Perspective*, 4th edn. Oxford: Wiley Blackwell. (This student textbook gives far more detail than the present book, but might be of interest for those wanting to pursue the subject); Gurr, M., Harwood, J., Frayn, K., Murphy, D., & Michell, R. (2016). *Lipids: Biochemistry, Biotechnology and Health*, 6th edn. Oxford: Wiley Blackwell. (This is a more specialised text. Some of the material in this chapter is based on it); Salway, J. G. (2017). *Metabolism at a Glance*, 4th edn. Oxford: Wiley Blackwell. (A clearly illustrated pictorial guide to metabolic pathways, aimed at undergraduate students).

More on fats: Pond, C. M. (1998). *The Fats of Life*. Cambridge: Cambridge University Press. (A readable account of the role of fats in the diet and in the body.)

On proteins: Protein Data Bank is a compendium of data on many proteins, showing the three-dimensional structure of the molecules in many cases. Insulin is at https://pdb101.rcsb.org/motm/14.

Chapter 3

Collins, J. M., Neville, M. J., Hoppa, M. B., & Frayn, K. N. (2010). *De novo* lipogenesis and stearoyl-CoA desaturase are coordinately regulated in the human adipocyte and protect against palmitate-induced cell injury. *J Biol Chem* 285: 6044–6052. (A research paper including an example of how molecules may be 'channelled' along a pathway.)

On metabolic pathway charts: Hadlington, S. (2007). *Life's Cartographer*. Chemistry World: www.chemistryworld.com/features/lifes-cartographer/3004664.article. (The personal story of Donald Nicholson, the man behind the chart of all known metabolic pathways); Nicholson, D. (2006). A lifetime of metabolism. *Cell Mol Life Sci* 63: 1–5. (Donald Nicholson's own story of how he created the first map of metabolic pathways.)

On the history of discovery of metabolic pathways: Fritz, I. B. (1961). Factors influencing the rates of long-chain fatty acid oxidation and synthesis in mammalian systems. *Physiol Rev* 41: 52–129 (an influential review for this author setting out to study lipid metabolism); Kresge, N., Simoni, R. D., & Hill, R. L. (2005). Fritz Lipmann and the discovery of coenzyme A. *J Biol Chem* 280: e18; Kresge, N., Simoni, R. D., & Hill, R. L. (2005). Otto Fritz Meyerhof and the elucidation of the glycolytic pathway. *J Biol Chem* 280: e3.

Chapter 4

BBC Bitesize: *Coordination and control – The nervous system.* www.bbc.co.uk/bitesize/guides/zprxy4j/revision/1 (a simple guide to the human nervous system).

Bliss, M. (1983). *The Discovery of Insulin.* Edinburgh: Paul Harris. (A very readable account of the early days in the story of insulin.)

On modification of enzyme activity by phosphorylation (adding a phosphate group to one of the protein's constituent amino acids): Cohen, P. (2009). Keep nibbling at the edges. *J Biol Chem* 284: 23891–23901 (Professor Sir Philip Cohen gives a personal account of the discovery of protein phosphorylation as a means of regulating enzyme activity); Cohen, P. (2021). Edmond Fischer (1920–2021). *Nature* 597: 328 (Philip Cohen's obituary for Edmond Fischer, one of the discoverers of protein phosphorylation to change enzyme activity, along with Edwin Krebs (not related to Hans Krebs): Fischer and Krebs were jointly awarded the Nobel Prize in Physiology or Medicine for their work in 1992).

Protein Data Bank: https://pdb101.rcsb.org/motm/14 (this web page shows the structure of insulin (shown in Figure 2.6) and discusses insulin's actions).

Robinson, A. M. & Williamson, D. H. (1980). Physiological roles of ketone bodies as substrates and signals in mammalian tissues. *Physiol Rev* 60: 143–187.

Sriram, K. & Insel, P. A. (2018). G protein-coupled receptors as targets for approved drugs: how many targets and how many drugs? *Mol Pharmacol* 93: 251–258. (This review highlights just how important the G protein-coupled receptors are for medicine development.)

Stallknecht, B., Lorentsen, J., Enevoldsen, L. H., Bülow, J., Biering-Sørensen, F., Galbo, H., & Kjaer, M. (2001). Role of the sympathoadrenergic system in adipose tissue metabolism during exercise in humans. *J Physiol* 536: 283–294.

Chapter 5

On mitochondria – origins and function: Friedman, J. R. & Nunnari, J. (2014). Mitochondrial form and function. *Nature* 505: 335–343; Newman, T. What are mitochondria? *Medical News Today.* Available at: www.medicalnewstoday.com/articles/320875

Guo, R., Gu, J., Zong, S., Wu, M. & Yang, M. (2018). Structure and mechanism of mitochondrial electron transport chain. *Biomed J* 41: 9–20. (In this open-access paper, Guo and colleagues describe what they term the 'respirasome', the complex of enzymes within the mitochondrion that brings about oxidation and ATP synthesis. It has clear pictures showing how the enzymes are arranged.)

Manzo-Avalos, S. & Saavedra-Molina, A. (2010). Cellular and mitochondrial effects of alcohol consumption. *Int J Environ Res Public Health* 7: 4281–4304. (An open-access paper giving more information about the metabolism of alcohol.)

Martinez-Reyes, I. & Chandel, N. S. (2020). Mitochondrial TCA cycle metabolites control physiology and disease. *Nat Commun* 11: 102. (A more in-depth open-access paper with information on the citric acid cycle (here called tricarboxylic acid, TCA, cycle).)

Nobel Prize in Chemistry (1978). www.nobelprize.org/prizes/chemistry/1978/sum mary/ (an account of Peter Mitchell's work on the chemiosmotic theory of ATP synthesis).

Chapter 6

Fery, F. D., Attellis, N. P., & Balasse, E. O. (1990). Mechanisms of starvation diabetes: study with double tracer and indirect calorimetry. *Am J Physiol* 259: E770–E777. (A research paper, not open access unfortunately but the abstract will give an idea how isotopic tracers can be used to study dynamic changes in metabolism following a meal (in this case, a glucose drink).)

On glucose and lactate inter-relationships: Brooks, G. A. (2020). Lactate as a fulcrum of metabolism. *Redox Biol* 35: 101454; Rabinowitz, J. D. & Enerbäck, S. (2020). Lactate: the ugly duckling of energy metabolism. *Nat Metab* 2: 566–571.

Kiela, P. R. & Ghishan, F. K. (2016). Physiology of intestinal absorption and secretion. *Best Pract Res Clin Gastroenterol* 30: 145–159. (An open-access review of this topic with much emphasis on micronutrients (such as vitamins) but also covering glucose, fats, and amino acids.)

On liver glucose metabolism: Petersen, M. C., Vatner, D. F., & Shulman, G. I. (2017). Regulation of hepatic glucose metabolism in health and disease. *Nat*

Rev Endocrinol 13: 572–587; Roach, P. J., Depaoli-Roach, A. A., Hurley, T. D. & Tagliabracci, V. S. (2012). Glycogen and its metabolism: some new developments and old themes. *Biochem J* 441: 763–787. (These are both open-access review papers giving detail about these systems in health and disease.)

On fat metabolism: Frayn, K. N., Arner, P. & Yki-Järvinen, H. (2006). Fatty acid metabolism in adipose tissue, muscle and liver in health and disease. *Essays Biochem* 42: 89–103.

Krebs, H. A. (1972). Some aspects of the regulation of fuel supply in omnivorous animals. *Adv Enz Reg* 10: 397–420. (Hans Krebs reflects especially on why amino acids are used as a metabolic fuel when present in excess.)

Valdes, A. M., Walter, J., Segal, E., & Spector, T. D. (2018). Role of the gut microbiota in nutrition and health. *BMJ* 361: k2179. (An accessible review on this topic.)

Yang, A. & Mottillo, E. P. (2020). Adipocyte lipolysis: from molecular mechanisms of regulation to disease and therapeutics. *Biochem J* 477: 985–1008 (open-access).

Chapter 7

On Adaptability Generally

Ashcroft, F. (2000). *Life at the Extremes: The Science of Survival*. London: Flamingo. (This readable book explores in more depth the adaptability of human physiology and metabolism.)

On Fasting

Benedict, F. G. (1915). *A Study of Prolonged Fasting*. Washington, DC: Carnegie Institute of Washington. Available via Forgotten Books: www.forgottenbooks.com/en/books/AStudyofProlongedFasting_10266160.

On the Minnesota experiment on semi-starvation: Kalm, L. M. & Semba, R. D. (2005). They starved so that others be better fed: remembering Ancel Keys and the Minnesota experiment. *J Nutr* 135: 1347–1352 (an account of Ancel Keys and the Minnesota Experiment on semi-starvation: not open-access but even the abstract will give you a feel for what was involved); Keys, A., Brožek, J., Henschel, A., Mickelsen, O., & Taylor, H. L. (1950). *The Biology of Human Starvation*, Volumes 1 & 2. Minneapolis, MN: University of Minnesota Press.

https://doi.org/10.5749/j.ctv9b2tqv; Tucker, T. (2008). *The Great Starvation Experiment: Ancel Keys and the Men Who Starved for Science*. Minneapolis, MN: University of Minnesota Press.

Owen, O. E., Morgan, A. P., Kemp, H. G., Sullivan, J. M., Herrera, M. G. & Cahill, G. F. (1967). Brain metabolism during fasting. *J Clin Invest* 46: 1589–1595.

Owen, O. E. (2005). Ketone bodies as a fuel for the brain during starvation. *Biochem Mol Biol Edu* 33: 246–251. (Oliver Owen's personal account of the classic studies on starvation of obese patients during the 1960s and later, under George Cahill.)

On Exercise and Stress

On different patterns of physical activity: Thompson, D., Karpe, F., Lafontan, M., & Frayn, K. (2012). Physical activity and exercise in the regulation of human adipose tissue physiology. *Physiol Rev* 92: 157–191; Thompson, D., Peacock, O., Western, M., & Batterham, A. M. (2015). Multidimensional physical activity: an opportunity, not a problem. *Exerc Sport Sci Rev* 43: 67–74.

Hawley, J. A., Maughan, R. J., & Hargreaves, M. (2015). Exercise metabolism: historical perspective. *Cell Metab* 22: 12–17. (An open-access review by three of the top scientists in exercise metabolism, giving a history of the field.)

On muscle metabolism in anaerobic exercise: Crowther, G. J., Carey, M. F., Kemper, W. F. & Conley, K. E. (2002). Control of glycolysis in contracting skeletal muscle. I. Turning it on. *Am J Physiol Endocrinol Metab* 282: E67–E73; Crowther, G. J., Kemper, W. F., Carey, M. F. & Conley, K. E. (2002). Control of glycolysis in contracting skeletal muscle. II. Turning it off. *Am J Physiol Endocrinol Metab* 282: E74–E79; Westerblad, H., Allen, D. G. & Lannergren, J. (2002). Muscle fatigue: lactic acid or inorganic phosphate the major cause? *News Physiol Sci* 17: 17–21.

On muscle glycogen and exercise: Bergström, J. & Hultman, E. (1966). Muscle glycogen synthesis after exercise: an enhancing factor localized to the muscle cells in man. *Nature* 210: 309–310 (the original observation of 'supercompensation'); Murray, B. & Rosenbloom, C. (2018). Fundamentals of glycogen metabolism for coaches and athletes. *Nutr Rev* 76: 243–259.

On fatty acids and stress: Frayn, K. N., Williams, C. M., & Arner, P. (1996). Are increased plasma non-esterified fatty acid concentrations a risk marker for coronary heart disease and other chronic diseases? *Clin Sci* 90: 243–253 (summarises the data behind the speculations about stress and heart disease). Newsholme, E. A. & Leech, A. R. (1983). *Biochemistry for the Medical Sciences*. Chichester: John Wiley (in this textbook the late British biochemist Eric Newsholme and his colleague Tony Leech present a detailed view of metabolism including speculations about fatty acids and stress. Their more recent book *Functional Biochemistry in Health and Disease* (Wiley-Blackwell, 2009) brings the biochemistry up to date but lacks some of the anecdotes).

Chapter 8

On how much we eat in 10 years: data taken from Public Health England/Food Standards Agency (2018). *National Diet and Nutrition Survey Results from Years 7 and 8 (combined) of the Rolling Programme (2014/2015 to 2015/2016)*. London: Crown Copyright.

Whitley, H. A., Humphreys, S. M., Samra, J. S., Campbell, I. T., Maclaren, D. P. M., Reilly, T. & Frayn, K. N. (1997). Metabolic responses to isoenergetic meals containing different proportions of carbohydrate and fat. *Br J Nutr* 78: 15–26.

On the physiological role of *de novo* lipogenesis: Acheson, K. J., Flatt, J. P., & Jéquier, E. (1982). Glycogen synthesis versus lipogenesis after a 500 gram carbohydrate meal in man. *Metabolism* 31: 1234–1240; Acheson, K. J., Schutz, Y., Bessard, T., Anantharaman, K., Flatt, J.-P. & Jéquier, E. (1988). Glycogen storage capacity and de novo lipogenesis during massive carbohydrate overfeeding in man. *Am J Clin Nutr* 48: 240–247.

King, R. F. G. J., Almond, D. J., Oxby, C. B., Holmfield, J. H. M., & McMahon, M. J. (1984). Calculation of short-term changes in body fat from measurement of respiratory gas exchange. *Metabolism* 33: 826–832.

On metabolic interactions between carbohydrates and fat: McGarry, J. D., Mannaerts, G. P., & Foster, D. W. (1977). A possible role for malonyl-CoA in the regulation of hepatic fatty acid oxidation and ketogenesis. *J Clin Invest* 60: 265–270; McGarry, J. D. (1979). Lilly Lecture 1978. New perspectives in the regulation of ketogenesis. *Diabetes* 28: 517–523; Randle, P. J., Garland, P. B., Hales, C. N., & Newsholme, E. A. (1963). The glucose fatty-acid cycle. Its role in insulin sensitivity and the metabolic disturbances of diabetes mellitus. *Lancet* 1: 785–789.

On longer-term regulation of gene expression by nutrients: Ferré, P. & Foufelle, F. (2007). SREBP-1c transcription factor and lipid homeostasis: clinical perspective. *Horm Res* 68: 72-82; González, A. & Hall, M. N. (2017). Nutrient sensing and TOR signaling in yeast and mammals. *EMBO J* 36: 397–408; Ortega-Prieto, P. & Postic, C. (2019). Carbohydrate sensing through the transcription factor ChREBP. *Front Genet* 10: 472.

Chapter 9

On genetics: Kampourakis, K. (2020). *Understanding Evolution*. Cambridge: Cambridge University Press; Kampourakis, K. (2022). *Understanding Genes*. Cambridge: Cambridge University Press.

On Mendelian inheritance of metabolic diseases: *Online Mendelian Inheritance in Man* (OMIM) is a free, online database (© Johns Hopkins University), and such disorders are often referred to be their OMIM catalogue number. Scriver's *The Online Metabolic & Molecular Bases of Inherited Disease* is a commercial catalogue.

On hereditability of leanness and obesity: Haworth, C. M., Plomin, R., Carnell, S., & Wardle, J. (2008). Childhood obesity: genetic and environmental overlap with normal-range BMI. *Obesity (Silver Spring)* 16: 1585–1590; Locke, A. E., Kahali, B., Berndt, S. I., et al. (2015). Genetic studies of body mass index yield new insights for obesity biology. *Nature* 518: 197–206.

On diabetes history and treatment: Bliss, M. (1983). *The Discovery of Insulin*. Edinburgh: Paul Harris; Mathieu, C., Martens, P. J., & Vangoitsenhoven, R. (2021). One hundred years of insulin therapy. *Nat Rev Endocrinol*. https://doi.org/10.1038/s41574-021-00542-w; Taylor, R., Al-Mrabeh, A., & Sattar, N. (2019). Understanding the mechanisms of reversal of type 2 diabetes. *Lancet Diabetes Endocrinol* 7: 726–736;

On cardiovascular disease mortality: Dagenais, G. R., Leong, D. P., Rangarajan, S., et al. (2020). Variations in common diseases, hospital admissions, and deaths in middle-aged adults in 21 countries from five continents (PURE): a prospective cohort study. *Lancet* 395: 785–794; WHO data: www.who.int/news-room/factsheets/detail/cardiovascular-diseases-(cvds).

On metabolism in cancer cells: Deberardinis, R. J. & Chandel, N. S. (2020). We need to talk about the Warburg effect. *Nat Metab* 2: 127–129; Swinnen, J. V., Brusselmans, K., & Verhoeven, G. (2006). Increased lipogenesis in cancer cells: new players, novel targets. *Curr Opin Clin Nutr Metab Care* 9: 358–365.

Figure Credits

Figure 1.2   From the Nobel Foundation Archive. www.nobelprize.org/prizes/medicine/1953/krebs/facts

Figure 2.1   Lower half reproduced from Frayn, K. N. & Evans, R. D. (2019). *Human Metabolism: A Regulatory Perspective*, 4th edn. Oxford: Wiley Blackwell, with permission from John Wiley & Sons, Inc.

Figure 2.2   Adapted from Gurr, M. I., Harwood, J. L., Frayn, K. N., Murphy, D. J. & Michell, R. H. (2016). *Lipids: Biochemistry, Biotechnology and Health*, 6th edn. Oxford: Wiley-Blackwell, with permission from John Wiley & Sons, Inc.

Figure 2.3   Reproduced from: https://commons.wikimedia.org/wiki/File:Triglyceride_unsaturated_Structural_Formulae_V.1.png

Figure 2.4   Reproduced from Frayn, K. N. & Evans, R. D. (2019). *Human Metabolism: A Regulatory Perspective*, 4th edn. Oxford: Wiley Blackwell, with permission from John Wiley & Sons, Inc.

Figure 2.5   Reproduced from Frayn, K. N. & Evans, R. D. (2019). *Human Metabolism: A Regulatory Perspective*, 4th edn. Oxford: Wiley Blackwell, with permission from John Wiley & Sons, Inc.

Figure 2.6   The insulin structure is from Goodsell, D. S. and RCSB Protein Data Bank; https://pdb101.rcsb.org/motm/14. Molecule of the Month: 10.2210/rcsb_pdb/mom_2001_2, reproduced under the Creative Commons Licence.

1080–1090. Republished with permission of the American Society for Clinical Investigation.

Figure 8.1 Modified from Whitley, H. A., Humphreys, S. M., Samra, J. S., Campbell, I. T., Maclaren, D. P. M., Reilly, T. & Frayn, K. N. (1997). Metabolic responses to isoenergetic meals containing different proportions of carbohydrate and fat. *British Journal of Nutrition* 78: 15–26. Reproduced with permission of Cambridge University Press.

Figure 8.2 © 2021, COSMED, Rome, Italy [www.cosmed.com] (with permission).

Figure 8.3 From Acheson, K. J., Schutz, Y., Bessard, T., Anantharaman, K., Flatt, J.-P. & Jéquier, E. (1988). Glycogen storage capacity and de novo lipogenesis during massive carbohydrate overfeeding in man. *American Journal of Clinical Nutrition* 48: 240–247. Republished with permission of the American Society for Nutrition.

Figure 8.5 The data are taken from Karpe, F., Fielding, B. A., Coppack, S. W., Lawrence, V. J., Macdonald, I. A. & Frayn, K. N. (2005). Oscillations of fatty acid and glycerol release from human subcutaneous adipose tissue in vivo. *Diabetes* 54: 1297–1303, and reproduced from Frayn, K. N. & Evans, R. D. (2019). *Human Metabolism: A Regulatory Perspective*, 4th edn. Oxford: Wiley Blackwell, with permission from John Wiley & Sons, Inc.

Figure 9.1 Reproduced from Bliss, M. (1983). *The Discovery of Insulin*. Edinburgh: Paul Harris.

Index

Printed in the United States
by Baker & Taylor Publisher Services